# WEIGHT MANAGEMENT SELF-HELP GUIDE

**U. S. DEPARTMENT
OF TRANSPORTATION**

**UNITED STATES
COAST GUARD**

**University Press of the Pacific
Honolulu, Hawaii**

Weight Management Self-Help Guide

by
United States Coast Guard

ISBN: 1-4101-0780-9

Copyright © 2005 by Fredonia Books

Reprinted from the 2002 edition

Fredonia Books
Amsterdam, The Netherlands
http://www.fredoniabooks.com

# Acknowledgments

This self-help guide was developed through a concerted effort of the United States Coast Guard Health Promotion Managers located at Integrated Support Command (ISC) Alameda, ISC Boston, ISC Cleveland, ISC Kodiak, ISC Honolulu, ISC Miami, ISC New Orleans, ISC Portsmouth, ISC St. Louis, ISC San Pedro, ISC Seattle, and Headquarters Support Command.

This guide was created to provide Coast Guard employees and their families assistance with managing their weight. While this guide is essentially self-explanatory, the maximum benefit and support can be realized by seeking the advice of your local Health Promotion Manager. This guide can be used by personnel who are voluntarily seeking to manage their weight, and by active duty members identified as exceeding their maximum allowable weight in accordance with Allowable Weight Standards for Coast Guard Military Personnel, COMDTINST M1020.8 (series).

You can contact your local Health Promotion Manager at your Regional Work-Life Staff. To contact the Work-Life Staff closest to you, call **1-800-872-4957**, followed by the extension listed next to the following **ISC locations**:

- *Alameda* (252)
- *Boston* (301)
- *Cleveland* (309)
- *Honolulu* (314)
- *Ketchikan* (317)
- *Kodiak* (563)
- *Miami* (307)
- *New Orleans* (308)
- *Portsmouth* (305)
- *San Pedro* (311)
- *Seattle* (313)
- *St. Louis* (302)
- *Mid-Atlantic* (932)

# TABLE OF CONTENTS

| TITLE | PAGE |
|---|---|

## Appendixes

# LIST OF WORKSHEETS

## List of Worksheets- continued

# LIST OF TABLES

## List of Tables- continued

# Introduction

# WHY DOES THE COAST GUARD CARE ABOUT WEIGHT MANAGEMENT?

## Overview

**Health Risk**

The National Institute of Health (NIH) has determined that a 20 percent increase above desirable body weight (as defined by NIH standards) substantially increases the risk for high blood pressure, heart disease, diabetes, elevated cholesterol and triglycerides. Obesity is also considered a risk factor for certain types of cancer and is associated with joint diseases, gallstones, and respiratory problems.

**Obesity**

According to statistics of the National Heart, Lung and Blood Institute (1999) 55 % of American adults are overweight and 22% are obese. *Obesity* is defined as an excessive accumulation of percent body fat. Obesity has become an enormous public health problem. (*Source*: http://rover.nhlbi.nih.gov/guidelines/obesity/ob_home.htm)

**Weight and Age**

Although many people in the United States gain weight with age, thus increasing their health risks, age itself is not a factor for weight gain. According to the 2000 Dietary Guidelines for Americans, it is recommended that we <u>not</u> allow our weight to increase as we age. Diseases associated with aging such as Type II diabetes, heart disease, and stroke are more prevalent in the obese population. (*Source:* http://www.ars.usda.gov/dgac/

**Exercise and Metabolism**

We tend to lose muscle and bone mass with age and increase percent of body fat. Metabolism slows about 5 percent every decade after age 30, therefore we must proportionately decrease food intake to remain balanced. We can slow down the effects of decreased metabolism and muscle mass *if we remain physically active.* Muscle tissue is metabolically more active than fat, therefore metabolism increases with gains in muscle tissue. A common myth is that weight gain increases with age. Studies indicate that weight gain is not primarily due to age but decreasing trends of physical activity in one's lifestyle.

**Fitness for Duty**

Fitness for duty is a critical element to Coast Guard mission accomplishment. Optimizing mission performance through enhanced physical well-being of all members is essential. In turn, this means assisting Coast Guard personnel to maintain healthy habits and a physically fit lifestyle. Maintaining healthy body weight and body composition (including percent fat) are elements of a fit lifestyle.

# Goal of this Workbook

> *The goal of this workbook is to provide you with the information, skills, and confidence to lose weight and maintain a healthy body composition and weight level.*

# Getting Started

**Self Responsibility**

Losing body fat and maintaining a healthy weight can be a difficult challenge. This requires making lifestyle changes with constant vigilance, commitment, and frequent self-evaluation. You may have setbacks from time to time. Acknowledging these setbacks and getting back on your program are half the battle. This self-guide is your first step.

There are various tools and methods available for weight management. There is no magic pill or easy approach to achieve a healthy lifestyle and maintain a healthy weight. The ultimate accomplishment of success is up to you. Your attitude and commitment are the critical factors for success.

This workbook is designed to be self-paced. It is a tool that provides information on basic nutrition, exercise concepts, and behavior modification to assist with safe weight loss and the maintenance of a healthy lifestyle. Whether or not you have access to professional nutritional guidance, this comprehensive guide is a useful tool to assist with successful weight loss and lifestyle management.

For additional support contact any of the following resources:

- *Unit Health Promotion Coordinator*
- *Regional Health Promotion Manager 1-800-USCGWLS*
- *CG Medical Officer for dietitian referral*
- *Employee Assistance Counselor 1-800-222-0364*

*Upon successful completion of this workbook you will be able to do the following:*

---

1.  ***Establish your realistic target weight and body fat composition.***

2.  ***Set a realistic time frame for your weight loss and/or body fat composition.***

3.  ***Calculate your appropriate caloric and nutritional intake.***

4.  ***Establish and modify your eating behaviors.***

5.  ***Establish and monitor your physical activity goals.***

6.  ***Identify and develop personal skills and support systems for a healthy lifestyle.***

---

**Basic Principles**  This workbook is based on the fundamental principles of weight management and behavioral change. A majority of commercial diet plans are actually very successful from the perspective that they do assist people in losing weight. However, studies show that 97% of people who subscribe to various fad diets, patronize weight loss clinics, or purchase expensive diet foods, regain their lost weight, and then some, within twelve months after stopping their program. With an emphasis on dietary balance, variety, physical exercise, and behavior modification you can be successful in maintaining your realistic and healthy weight level. Weight loss is not the primary challenge; rather the ultimate challenge is weight maintenance.

**Table I-1.  Principles of Successful Weight Management**

---

- Adopt eating habits that support a lifelong behavior.

- Weight management requires an ongoing commitment on your part and a realization that it is going to take time.

- Increase physical activity and exercise to expend additional calories.

- Successful change requires applying behavior modification techniques.

- Goal setting is essential, but weight loss is not the goal.

- A restrictive diet is not recommended. A healthy diet follows the concepts of balance, variety, and moderation, such as the recommendations of the American Heart Association and the Food Guide Pyramid.

- Learn to handle stress without using food as a reward or punishment.

- Use food solely to meet physical nutritional requirements, not emotional needs.

- Learn to cook in a healthier manner.

- 1200 calories per day is the minimum needed to obtain the necessary nutrients for a healthy diet.

---

**The *Diet* Mentality**

The word "diet" implies going on a temporary plan.  It also implies being restricted from eating certain foods. These are two main reasons people "on diets" fail to maintain weight loss. Many people lose weight easily, but find it more difficult to keep if off.  A lifestyle that includes a **healthy eating plan** and **regular physical activity** will lead to and maintain a healthier you. This is the key.  Keeping weight off depends on your commitment to a lifestyle change.

## The Role of Metabolism

A person's total daily caloric output is determined by the sum of the energy required in:

- *Resting metabolism*
- *Thermal effect of food*
- *Physical activity*

## What is Metabolism?

*Metabolism* is defined by scientists as the chemical reactions that make the energy in foods available to the various physiological systems of the body. For instance, energy is required for muscular activity, the growth of skin, hair, nails, maintenance of body temperature, and even the digestion of food. A way to measure the rate of metabolism is to measure the rate at which the body uses oxygen. This is called *basal metabolic rate*, or simply BMR (*basal metabolic rate* and *resting metabolic rate* are used interchangeably). Metabolism acts as the body's thermostat, much like the thermostat in your house. BMR accounts for approximately 60-75 percent of daily caloric output.

## Influence of Body Size

Body size affects resting metabolism. BMR is proportional to the surface area of the body. This means that *larger individuals burn more calories than smaller individuals for similar activities.* Differences in body composition also affect BMR. Fat tissue is metabolically less active than muscle or lean body mass. Athletes with greater muscle development show a greater increase in metabolism over the non-athlete. Muscle accounts for approximately 20 percent of resting metabolism. Women, who tend to have more fat in proportion to muscle than men, have metabolic rates 5-10 percent lower than men of the same weight and height. When based on the same amount of lean body mass, metabolic rates for men and women are similar. The same phenomenon is observed with aging. In general, as people age, lean body mass decreases and fat mass increases. A 5 percent decrease in BMR with every 10 years of life is usually observed through adulthood.

## The Effect of BMR

BMR affects weight management because the overweight person who carries too much body fat and not enough lean muscle mass has a slower BMR. Therefore, getting leaner will help boost your BMR. How do we change the ratio of fat to muscle? Some commercial programs claim that we can turn fat into muscle and vice versa. This is **not** true. Fat tissues are round receptacles designed to store fat. Excess calories in the diet causes fat cells to grow in size as they store more fat. Conversely, fat cells shrink when you burn more calories than you eat. Thus fat cells never disappear, they simply shrink. Muscle fibers increase in size when worked (hypertrophy), and muscle fibers decrease in size when not used (atrophy).

## Thermal Effects of Food

Eating, due to the energy-requiring process of digesting, absorbing, and metabolizing the various nutrients, stimulates an increase in metabolic rate. This accounts for approximately 10 percent of total caloric output. This process is sometimes referred to as the "specific dynamic action" or "dietary-induced thermogenesis." It reaches a maximum within 1 hour after a meal. Skipping meals tends to decrease metabolic rate so you burn calories at a lower rate (in other words, you lower your thermostat). Not eating enough can be as bad as eating too much! (This concept is discussed more in Chapter 4).

**Effects of Physical Activity**

Physical activity can have the most profound effect on caloric output. On average, physical activity accounts for 15-30 percent of total caloric output. Most of us can generate substantial increases in metabolism (up to 10 times the resting value) during sustained exercise such as running or cycling. The bottom line is *the more physically active the person is, the higher his/her metabolism will be.*

# The Energy Balance Equation for Weight Management

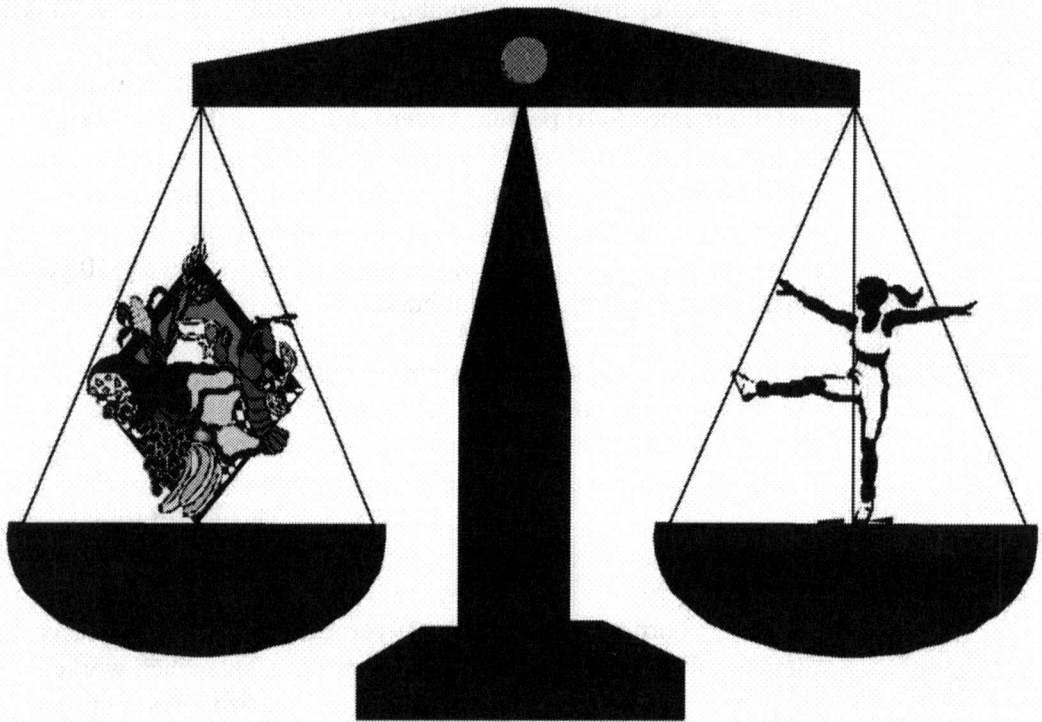

**ENERGY IN**          **=**          **ENERGY OUT**

*Food (Calories)*                    *Caloric Output*
*Proteins*                             *Resting Metabolism*
*Carbohydrates*                   *Food Digestion*
*Fats*                                    *Physical Activity*

# Chapter 1

# DEVELOPING AN ACTION PLAN

## Overview

Now that you have considered all of the essential elements of successful weight management, it's time to put together an ACTION PLAN. **Worksheet 1-1** will help you do this. *In order to complete all of the steps in your action plan, you will first need to answer the assessment, and worksheets in this Guide.* They will help you identify the specific steps in your ACTION PLAN.

Most importantly, your plan needs to be *realistic and relevant* to *you*. Remember that this is YOUR plan. Studies clearly show that people who set objectives, develop an action plan, and keep records are more successful at meeting and maintaining their weight management goals. Your plan is like a road map; when you plan a trip you use a road map to guide you to your destination. Your ACTION PLAN is your roadmap to reach your goals. It is the map for your journey toward better health.

## Worksheet 1-1. My Weight Management Plan

*This worksheet outlines the necessary steps for successful weight management. In order to establish this plan you will need to complete the assessment and worksheet referred to in each step. If more space is needed to complete a step refer back to the accompanying worksheet.*

### Step 1. My Top Motivators.

*(See Worksheet 1-3, page 1-5)*

a. _____

b. _____

### Step 2. My Weight Management Objective.

*(See Worksheet 1-4, page 1-6)*

_____

_____

**My Weight
Management
Plan (cont.)**

## Step 3. My Weight and Body Fat Composition Targets.

*(See Tables 2-2 & 2-3, page 2-2, or Worksheet 2-1, page 2-6)*

a. Target weight: _____ pounds

b. Target body fat composition: _____ %.

## Step 4. My Realistic Time Frame.

*(See Worksheet 3-1, page 3-2)*

Target weight loss date: _____

## Step 5. My Daily Calorie and Fat Intake Goal.

*(See Worksheet 4-1, page 4-6 & Worksheet 4-2, page 4-9)*

a. Caloric need: _____ calories/day

b. Adjusted fat budget: _____ grams/day

## Step 6. My Personal Nutrition Plan.

*(See Worksheet 4-7, page 4-35)*

a. Prudent nutrition strategies: _____

b. Calorie control strategies: _____

c. Reducing fat intake: _____

d. Reducing sodium: _____

# Worksheet 1-1.  My Weight Management Plan (cont.)

**My Weight Management Plan (cont.)**

## Step 7. My Modified Eating Patterns.

*(See Worksheet 5-7, page 5-11, Worksheet 5-8, page 5-12, Worksheet 6-1, page 6-2, Worksheet 6-2, page 6-2, Worksheet 7-1, page 7-1)*

    a.  Changing my food cues: _____

    b.  Planning new eating behaviors: _____

    c.  Healthy galley menu choices: _____

    d.  Galley low-calorie choices: _____

    e.  New dining-out behaviors: _____

## Step 8. My Physical Activity (FITT) Plan.

*(See Worksheet 8-3, page 8-13, & Worksheet 8-5, page 8-15)*

    a.  Frequency: _____

    b.  Days of the week: Mon. Tues. Wed. Thurs. Fri. Sat. Sun.

    c.  Calories Expended per exercise session _____calories

    d.  Intensity (THR Zone): _____ bpm

    e.  Time (length) of exercise session: _____ minutes

    f.  Type of Activity: _____

## Step 9. My Lifestyle Changes to Support My Weight Management.

*(See Worksheet 9-2, page 9-10)*

    a.  Stress management techniques: _____

    b.  Change self-talk: _____

    c.  Recognize & reward success: _____

    d.  Seek personal & social support: _____

    e.  Assert my needs: _____

Signed: _____ Date _____

Witness (*optional*) _____ Date _____

**Motivating Factors**

## Worksheet 1-2.  Motivating Factors to Lose Weight

*First, check the reasons listed below that are important to your decision. If your most important reasons aren't included, add them to the list. Second, assign a ranking for the reasons you have checked (1 is most important, etc.).*

|  | Important (Y/N) | Ranking |
|---|---|---|
| 1. Follow my doctor's advice | \_\_\_\_\_ | \_\_\_\_\_ |
| 2. Wear a smaller clothing size | \_\_\_\_\_ | \_\_\_\_\_ |
| 3. Improve my appearance | \_\_\_\_\_ | \_\_\_\_\_ |
| 4. Feel more assured | \_\_\_\_\_ | \_\_\_\_\_ |
| 5. Feel healthier | \_\_\_\_\_ | \_\_\_\_\_ |
| 6. Feel more in control of myself | \_\_\_\_\_ | \_\_\_\_\_ |
| 7. Strengthen and tone muscle | \_\_\_\_\_ | \_\_\_\_\_ |
| 8. Please someone who is important to me | \_\_\_\_\_ | \_\_\_\_\_ |
| 9. Improve sports performance or increase physical activity | \_\_\_\_\_ | \_\_\_\_\_ |
| 10. Help reduce low-back pain | \_\_\_\_\_ | \_\_\_\_\_ |
| 11. Reduce a health risk (specify) _____ | \_\_\_\_\_ | \_\_\_\_\_ |
| 12. Have more energy and increase stamina | \_\_\_\_\_ | \_\_\_\_\_ |
| 13. Meet the CG Weight Standards | \_\_\_\_\_ | \_\_\_\_\_ |
| 14. Other _____ | \_\_\_\_\_ | \_\_\_\_\_ |

**Motivating Factors**

# <u>Worksheet 1-3. Top Motivators</u>

*For your top two reasons write out why these are your most important and how you think these reasons will help motivate you to start and maintain your weight management program.*

#1 is _____. This is important because _____

_____

#2 is _____. This is important because _____

_____

*<u>Now, go back to page 1-1 and complete Step 1 on Worksheet 1-1, My Weight Management Plan.</u>*

**Samples of Goals**

The table below lists a number of general nutrition, fitness, and stress-management goals to assist in identifying your own goals. Check the ones that are important to your weight management plan. You can then design SMART objectives to help you meet your goals.

## <u>Table 1-1. Sample Goals</u>

| | | | |
|---|---|---|---|
| ? | Read food labels when buying foods. | ? | Select one or more physical activities to perform three-five times weekly. |
| ? | Modify food servings/ portion sizes. | ? | Improve heart and lung (cardiorespiratory) fitness. |
| ? | Eat at least 5 servings of fruits & vegetables daily. | ? | Improve muscular strength & endurance. |
| ? | Include foods that are good sources of calcium. | ? | Improve flexibility. |
| ? | Drink plenty of water- at least 64 oz. daily (8 glasses). | ? | Walk vs. taking the car whenever possible. |
| ? | Reduce total fat intake to 30% or less, with saturated fats to 10%. | ? | Practice a structured relaxation technique at least 3 times a week. |
| ? | Use the Food Pyramid as a guideline for meal planning. | ? | Incorporate laughter & humor into daily lifestyle. |
| ? | Increase dietary fiber intake to 30 grams a day. | ? | Include *quality* social interaction on a daily basis. |
| ? | Other: | ? | Other: |

## Setting a S.M.A.R.T. Objective

As you go through the process of changing and adopting healthy habits, you are actively taking charge of your health. Begin by setting objectives that are **SMART**- Specific, Measurable, Action-oriented, Realistic and Timed. Here is a brief description of each SMART element.

- **Specific** - The more specific, the easier it is to plan your routines to reach your goal. For example, rather than stating " I want to increase my dietary fiber intake" you would restate "I will add one additional serving each of fruits and vegetables to my daily diet."

- **Measurable** - Your objective should be easy to measure so you can chart your progress. Taking the fiber example from above, you can record your fruit and vegetable intake and track your progress.

- **Action-oriented** - State exactly what actions you must do to achieve your goal. For example, "Today I will eat a banana for an afternoon snack."

- **Realistic** - Be realistic in your expectations of yourself and what you hope to accomplish. It is important to identify and change unrealistic weight-loss objective you may have set for yourself because unrealistic objectives set you up for failure. Take large or long-term goals and break them into smaller, more manageable objectives. For example, plan to add one additional serving of fruit and vegetables a week for the first two weeks. Increase the serving amounts until you have reached the objective of one additional daily serving.

- **Timed** - Time lines let you know where you are along the journey. They are a way of marking progress with your objectives to reach your long-term goal. Using the dietary fiber example, this would mean increasing your weekly serving intake every two weeks -- for a total of fourteen weeks.

Here is a sample weight management objective:

*By April 15th I will be within the Coast Guard Weight Standards by two percent. I will accomplish this by decreasing my daily caloric intake by 250 calories and by increasing my exercise activity to expend an additional 250 calories each day.*

**My Weight Management Objective**

## Worksheet 1-4.  My Weight Management Objective

_____

_____

*Now, go back to page 1-1 and complete Step 2 on Worksheet 1-1, My Weight Management Plan.*

# Chapter 2

# DETERMINING YOUR TARGET WEIGHT AND BODY FAT

## Overview

There are a number of ways you can determine your realistic and healthy body weight and body fat. Three methods are presented here:

*A. Height-weight chart*
*B. Body Mass Index (BMI) table*
*C. Calculating target body weight and body fat composition.*

**Height-Weight Standards**

*Table 2-2 and 2-3 represents optimal weight for fitness, health, and uniform appearance for most people (Source: Metropolitan Life Insurance). Before you can check to see if your weight is optimal for your height and gender you need to determine your frame size.*

**Frame Size**

If you have always wondered what size frame you are, here is the method that corresponds with the Table 2-1. This will be easier with the help of a friend.

1. Extend your arm in front of your body bending your elbow at a ninety-degree angle to your body (finger tips face the ceiling). Your arm is parallel to your body.

2. Keep your fingers straight and turn the inside of your wrist to your body.

3. Place your thumb and index finger on the two prominent bones on either side of your elbow, measure the distance between the bones with a tape measure.

4. Compare to the medium-framed chart below. Select your height based on what you are barefoot. If you are below the listed inches, your frame is small. If you are above, your frame is large.

## Table 2-1. Frame Size

*Elbow Measurements for Medium Frame Size*

| Height in 1" heels | Elbow | Height in 1" heels | Elbow |
|---|---|---|---|
| **Men** | Breadth | **Women** | Breadth |
| 5'2"-5'3" | 2 1/2"-2 7/8" | 4'10"-4'11" | 2 1/4"-2 1/2" |
| 5'4"-5'7" | 2 5/8"-2 7/8" | 5'0"-5'3" | 2 1/4"-2 1/2" |
| 5'8"-5'11" | 2 3/4"-3" | 5'4"-5'7" | 2 3/8"-2 5/8" |
| 6'0"-6'3" | 2 3/4"-3 1/8" | 5'8"-5'11" | 2 3/8"-2 5/8" |
| 6'4" | 2 7/8"-3 1/4" | 6'0" | 2 1/2"-2 3/4" |

# Table 2-2. Height-Weight Chart

**Height-Weight Standards**

- **Height & Weight Table For Women**

| Height Feet Inches | Small Frame | Medium Frame | Large Frame |
|---|---|---|---|
| 4' 10" | 102-111 | 109-121 | 118-131 |
| 4' 11" | 103-113 | 111-123 | 120-134 |
| 5' 0" | 104-115 | 113-126 | 122-137 |
| 5' 1" | 106-118 | 115-129 | 125-140 |
| 5' 2" | 108-121 | 118-132 | 128-143 |
| 5' 3" | 111-124 | 121-135 | 131-147 |
| 5' 4" | 114-127 | 124-138 | 134-151 |
| 5' 5" | 117-130 | 127-141 | 137-155 |
| 5' 6" | 120-133 | 130-144 | 140-159 |
| 5' 7" | 123-136 | 133-147 | 143-163 |
| 5' 8" | 126-139 | 136-150 | 146-167 |
| 5' 9" | 129-142 | 139-153 | 149-170 |
| 5' 10" | 132-145 | 142-156 | 152-173 |
| 5' 11" | 135-148 | 145-159 | 155-176 |
| 6' 0" | 138-151 | 148-162 | 158-179 |

Weights at ages 25-59 based on lowest mortality. Weight in pounds according to frame (in indoor clothing weighing 3 lbs.; shoes with 1" heels)

- **Height & Weight Table For Men**

| Height Feet Inches | Small Frame | Medium Frame | Large Frame |
|---|---|---|---|
| 5' 2" | 128-134 | 131-141 | 138-150 |
| 5' 3" | 130-136 | 133-143 | 140-153 |
| 5" 4" | 132-138 | 135-145 | 142-156 |
| 5' 5" | 134-140 | 137-148 | 144-160 |
| 5' 6" | 136-142 | 139-151 | 146-164 |
| 5' 7" | 138-145 | 142-154 | 149-168 |
| 5' 8" | 140-148 | 145-157 | 152-172 |
| 5' 9" | 142-151 | 148-160 | 155-176 |
| 5' 10" | 144-154 | 151-163 | 158-180 |
| 5' 11" | 146-157 | 154-166 | 161-184 |
| 6' 0" | 149-160 | 157-170 | 164-188 |
| 6' 1" | 152-164 | 160-174 | 168-192 |
| 6' 2" | 155-168 | 164-178 | 172-197 |
| 6' 3" | 158-172 | 167-182 | 176-202 |
| 6' 4" | 162-176 | 171-187 | 181-207 |

Weights at ages 25-59 based on lowest mortality. Weight in pounds according to frame (in indoor clothing weighing 5 lbs.; shoes with 1" heels)

# Table 2-3. Body Mass Index (BMI)

*This is a rough measure of body composition that is useful if you don't have access to body composition testing. Though more accurate than height-weight tables, BMI is based on the concept that weight should be proportional to height. A healthy BMI range is 19-25. Use the following tables to determine your BMI*

## Body Mass Index Table

To use the table, find the appropriate height in the left-hand column. Move across to a given weight. The number at the top of the column is the BMI at that height and weight. Pounds have been rounded off.

| BMI | 19 | 20 | 21 | 22 | 23 | 24 | 25 | 26 | 27 | 28 | 29 | 30 | 31 | 32 | 33 | 34 | 35 | 36 |
|---|---|---|---|---|---|---|---|---|---|---|---|---|---|---|---|---|---|---|
| Height inches | Body Weight (pounds) | | | | | | | | | | | | | | | | | |
| 58 | 91 | 96 | 100 | 105 | 110 | 115 | 119 | 124 | 129 | 134 | 138 | 143 | 148 | 153 | 158 | 162 | 167 | 172 |
| 59 | 94 | 99 | 104 | 109 | 114 | 119 | 124 | 128 | 133 | 138 | 143 | 148 | 153 | 158 | 163 | 168 | 173 | 178 |
| 60 | 97 | 102 | 107 | 112 | 118 | 123 | 128 | 133 | 138 | 143 | 148 | 153 | 158 | 163 | 168 | 174 | 179 | 184 |
| 61 | 100 | 106 | 111 | 116 | 122 | 127 | 132 | 137 | 143 | 148 | 153 | 158 | 164 | 169 | 174 | 180 | 185 | 190 |
| 62 | 104 | 109 | 115 | 120 | 126 | 131 | 136 | 142 | 147 | 153 | 158 | 164 | 169 | 175 | 180 | 186 | 191 | 196 |
| 63 | 107 | 113 | 118 | 124 | 130 | 135 | 141 | 146 | 152 | 158 | 163 | 169 | 175 | 180 | 186 | 191 | 197 | 203 |
| 64 | 110 | 116 | 122 | 128 | 134 | 140 | 145 | 151 | 157 | 163 | 169 | 174 | 180 | 186 | 192 | 197 | 204 | 209 |
| 65 | 114 | 120 | 126 | 132 | 138 | 144 | 150 | 156 | 162 | 168 | 174 | 180 | 186 | 192 | 198 | 204 | 210 | 216 |
| 66 | 118 | 124 | 130 | 136 | 142 | 148 | 155 | 161 | 167 | 173 | 179 | 186 | 192 | 198 | 204 | 210 | 216 | 223 |
| 67 | 121 | 127 | 134 | 140 | 146 | 153 | 159 | 166 | 172 | 178 | 185 | 191 | 198 | 204 | 211 | 217 | 223 | 230 |
| 68 | 125 | 131 | 138 | 144 | 151 | 158 | 164 | 171 | 177 | 184 | 190 | 197 | 203 | 210 | 216 | 223 | 230 | 236 |
| 69 | 128 | 135 | 142 | 149 | 155 | 162 | 169 | 176 | 182 | 189 | 196 | 203 | 209 | 216 | 223 | 230 | 236 | 243 |
| 70 | 132 | 139 | 146 | 153 | 160 | 167 | 174 | 181 | 188 | 195 | 202 | 209 | 216 | 222 | 229 | 236 | 243 | 250 |
| 71 | 136 | 143 | 150 | 157 | 165 | 172 | 179 | 186 | 193 | 200 | 208 | 215 | 222 | 229 | 236 | 243 | 250 | 257 |
| 72 | 140 | 147 | 154 | 162 | 169 | 177 | 184 | 191 | 199 | 206 | 213 | 221 | 228 | 235 | 242 | 250 | 258 | 265 |
| 73 | 144 | 151 | 159 | 166 | 174 | 182 | 189 | 197 | 204 | 212 | 219 | 227 | 235 | 242 | 250 | 257 | 265 | 272 |
| 74 | 148 | 155 | 163 | 171 | 179 | 186 | 194 | 202 | 210 | 218 | 225 | 233 | 241 | 249 | 256 | 264 | 272 | 280 |
| 75 | 152 | 160 | 168 | 176 | 184 | 192 | 200 | 208 | 216 | 224 | 232 | 240 | 248 | 256 | 264 | 272 | 279 | 287 |
| 76 | 156 | 164 | 172 | 180 | 189 | 197 | 205 | 213 | 221 | 230 | 238 | 246 | 254 | 263 | 271 | 279 | 287 | 295 |

**Classifications: Underweight:** less than 19; **Normal:** 19-25; **Overweight:** 25-30; **Obesity I:** 30-35; **Obesity II:** 35-40; **Obesity III:** Over 40

(*Source: National Heart, Lung and Blood Institute, 1998*)

# Table 2-3. Body Mass Index (BMI) (cont.)

**Body Mass Index Table**

To use the table, find the appropriate height in the left-hand column. Move across to a given weight. The number at the top of the column is the BMI at that height and weight. Pounds have been rounded off.

| BMI / Height inches | 37 | 38 | 39 | 40 | 41 | 42 | 43 | 44 | 45 | 46 | 47 | 48 | 49 | 50 | 51 | 52 | 53 | 54 |
|---|---|---|---|---|---|---|---|---|---|---|---|---|---|---|---|---|---|---|
| | | | | | | | | | Body Weight (pounds) | | | | | | | | | |
| 58 | 177 | 181 | 186 | 191 | 196 | 201 | 205 | 210 | 215 | 220 | 224 | 229 | 234 | 239 | 244 | 248 | 253 | 258 |
| 59 | 183 | 188 | 193 | 198 | 203 | 208 | 212 | 217 | 222 | 227 | 232 | 237 | 242 | 247 | 252 | 257 | 262 | 267 |
| 60 | 189 | 194 | 199 | 204 | 209 | 215 | 220 | 225 | 230 | 235 | 240 | 245 | 250 | 255 | 261 | 266 | 271 | 276 |
| 61 | 195 | 201 | 206 | 211 | 217 | 222 | 227 | 232 | 238 | 243 | 248 | 254 | 259 | 264 | 269 | 275 | 280 | 285 |
| 62 | 202 | 207 | 213 | 218 | 224 | 229 | 235 | 240 | 246 | 251 | 256 | 262 | 267 | 273 | 278 | 284 | 289 | 295 |
| 63 | 208 | 214 | 220 | 225 | 231 | 237 | 242 | 248 | 254 | 259 | 265 | 270 | 278 | 282 | 287 | 293 | 299 | 304 |
| 64 | 215 | 221 | 227 | 232 | 238 | 244 | 250 | 256 | 262 | 267 | 273 | 279 | 285 | 291 | 296 | 302 | 308 | 314 |
| 65 | 222 | 228 | 234 | 240 | 246 | 252 | 258 | 264 | 270 | 275 | 282 | 288 | 294 | 300 | 306 | 312 | 318 | 324 |
| 66 | 229 | 235 | 241 | 247 | 253 | 260 | 266 | 272 | 278 | 284 | 291 | 297 | 303 | 309 | 315 | 322 | 328 | 334 |
| 67 | 236 | 242 | 249 | 255 | 261 | 268 | 274 | 280 | 287 | 293 | 299 | 306 | 312 | 319 | 325 | 331 | 338 | 344 |
| 68 | 243 | 249 | 256 | 262 | 269 | 276 | 282 | 289 | 295 | 302 | 308 | 315 | 322 | 328 | 335 | 341 | 348 | 354 |
| 69 | 250 | 257 | 263 | 270 | 277 | 284 | 291 | 297 | 304 | 311 | 318 | 324 | 331 | 338 | 345 | 351 | 358 | 365 |
| 70 | 257 | 264 | 271 | 278 | 285 | 292 | 299 | 306 | 313 | 320 | 327 | 334 | 341 | 348 | 355 | 362 | 369 | 376 |
| 71 | 265 | 272 | 279 | 286 | 293 | 301 | 308 | 315 | 322 | 329 | 338 | 343 | 351 | 358 | 365 | 372 | 379 | 386 |
| 72 | 272 | 279 | 287 | 294 | 302 | 309 | 316 | 324 | 331 | 338 | 346 | 353 | 361 | 368 | 375 | 383 | 390 | 397 |
| 73 | 280 | 288 | 295 | 302 | 310 | 318 | 325 | 333 | 340 | 348 | 355 | 363 | 371 | 378 | 386 | 393 | 401 | 408 |
| 74 | 287 | 295 | 303 | 311 | 319 | 326 | 334 | 342 | 350 | 358 | 365 | 373 | 381 | 389 | 396 | 404 | 412 | 420 |
| 75 | 295 | 303 | 311 | 319 | 327 | 335 | 343 | 351 | 359 | 367 | 375 | 383 | 391 | 399 | 407 | 415 | 423 | 431 |
| 76 | 304 | 312 | 320 | 328 | 336 | 344 | 353 | 361 | 369 | 377 | 385 | 394 | 402 | 410 | 418 | 426 | 435 | 443 |

**Classifications: Underweight:** less than 19; **Normal:** 19-25; **Overweight:** 25-30; **Obesity I:** 30-35; **Obesity II:** 35-40; **Obesity III:** Over 40

*(Source: National Heart, Lung and Blood Institute, 1998)*

2-4

# Assessing Body Fat Composition

**Overview**

Body fat includes both essential and non-essential fats. Essential fat includes lipids that are incorporated into the nerves, brain, heart, lungs, liver, and mammary glands. Nonessential (storage) fat exists primarily within fat cells, or adipose tissue, often located just below the skin and around major organs (which is visceral fat). Excess storage fat is usually the result of consuming more calories than is expended.

Most importantly, for health and weight loss is the body's total fat weight - the percentage body fat to the lean mass. Too much body fat has negative effects on health and well being.

- *Overweight* is usually defined as the total weight above the recommended range for age height, and gender.

- *Obesity* is defined as an excessive accumulation of body fat. These standards vary, depending on health status and the presence of other risk factors. For example, a person with high blood pressure and high cholesterol may want to reduce percentage of body fat, even if it is within the acceptable range.

**Negative Health Consequences**

An obese person is at increased risk for the following health problems:

| | |
|---|---|
| • Early death | • Complications during pregnancy |
| • Cardiovascular disease | • Menstrual abnormalities |
| • Hypertension | • Diabetes |
| • Gallbladder disease | • Heart Attack & Stroke |
| • Cancer | • Shortness of breath |
| • Back Pain | • Arthritis & Gout |
| • Elevated Cholesterol | • Impaired Heart Function |

**Body Fat Composition**

Your body fat composition can be measured by your regional Health Program Manager or at a local fitness center. If your regional Health Promotion Manager or local fitness center assesses your body composition it does not replace your body fat measurement for the Allowable Weight Standards for Coast Guard Military Personnel, COMDTINST M1020.8 (series).

## Table 2-4. Percent Body Fat Classifications

| Classification | Men | Women |
|---|---|---|
| Excessively Lean | 5% or less | 8% or less |
| Lean | 5-11% | 8-19% |
| Acceptable | 12-20% | 20-30% |
| Borderline Obese | 21-25% | 31-33% |
| Obese | Over 25% | Over 33% |

*Source: The Cooper Institute for Aerobics Research, Dallas TX.*

**Target Body Fat and Weight**

## Worksheet 2-1. Calculating Target Body Fat and Weight

These steps are a more specific method for calculating your target body weight and body fat percentage. *In order to use this method you must know your current body fat percentage.* Make arrangements with your regional Health Promotion Manager to have a body composition assessment.

1. Your Current Body Weight (**CBW**)          _____

   *Example: 200 lbs.*

2. Your **Current** Body Fat Composition in (**% CBF**)    _____

   Use decimal format  *Example: 25% = .25*

3. Determine **Target** Body Composition in (**% TBC**)    _____

   Refer to Table 2-3. Percent Body Fat Classification

   *Example: 20% BF for 35 yr. old male (Acceptable level)*

**Calculating Body Fat and Weight**

4. Calculate **Current** Fat Weight (**CFW**)  _____

   Multiply **CBW** (Step 1) x **CBF%** (Step 2) in decimal format

   *Example: 200 lbs. x .25 = 50 lbs.*

5. Calculate Current Lean Body Weight (**CLW**)  _____

   Subtract **CFW** (Step 4) from **CBW** (Step 1)

   *Example: 200 lbs. - 50 lbs. = 150 lbs.*

6. Calculate **Target** Lean Weight Percentage (**TLW%**):  _____

   Subtract **TBC%** (Step 3) from 100% in decimal format

   *Example: 100% (1.00) - 20% (.20) = 80% (.80)*

7. Calculate TARGET WEIGHT **(TW)**  _____

   **(TW)** by dividing **CLW** (Step 5) by **TLW%** (Step 6)

   *Example: 150 lbs/.80 = 187.5 lbs.*

8. *Calculate POUNDS NEEDED TO LOSE*  _____

   Subtract **TW** (Step 7) from **CBW** (Step 1)

   *Example: 200 lbs. – 187.5 lbs. = 12.5 lbs.*

**Frame Size**

Since we have not made an allowance for frame size (small, medium, or large), this "target weight" may not be the weight that you want to achieve.  You may need to weigh a little more or a little less depending on your frame size (generally, 10 percent is subtracted for small frame, and 10 percent is added for large frame individuals).

***Now, go back to page 1-2 and complete Step 3 on Worksheet 1-1, My Weight Management Plan.***

# Chapter 3

# TRACKING YOUR WEIGHT LOSS

## Overview

**What's a Reasonable Weight Loss Rate?**

The combination of decreased calories and increased physical activity provide the most effective way to lose weight. *Safe weight loss is one-half to two pounds per week for the average person.* Some weight loss plans claim you can lose five or more pounds in a week. Such rapid weight loss is likely to be fluid loss and not true fat loss. Don't be fooled by these claims!

**To Weigh or Not to Weigh?**

The scale can be your best friend or your worst enemy. Weighing yourself is an important monitoring tool, as long as you keep it in proper perspective. Your weight on a scale can vary throughout the day and from scale to scale. <u>How often</u> you need to weigh yourself is left up to your interpretation; the general rule is once a week.

Many people practice the unhealthy habit of "scale avoidance." Experts agree that you can become "blind" to weight increases. Keep in mind the scale cannot tell the difference between you and a sack of potatoes. Likewise, the scale cannot tell muscle mass from fat mass (the average Mr. Olympia weighs 300 pounds). Circumference measurements are the most reliable in telling differences in body composition (fat mass vs. muscle mass), as inches lost are usually more significant than pounds lost. Muscle mass weighs more than fat mass, but it takes up less space on your body.

To ensure consistent results, try to weigh yourself on the same scale, with the same amount of clothing or naked, at the same time of day.

**Charting Your Weight Management Goal**

A helpful way to track your weight management goals is to maintain a WEIGHT MANAGEMENT CHART. The worksheet on the following page will assist you with this method.

# Worksheet 3-1.  Charting Weight Management

Starting weight _____      Starting Date _____

Target Weight _____      Target Date _____

**_Now, go to page 1-2 and complete Step 4 on Worksheet 1-1, My Weight Management Plan._**

*The following chart will help you monitor your progress. Weigh yourself once a week on the same day. Compare that weight to your starting weight. Then place an "X" in the box that corresponds to your loss or gain for the week. Draw a line between each week's results. This will give you a graph to help visualize your progress.*

## WEIGHT MANAGEMENT PROGRESS

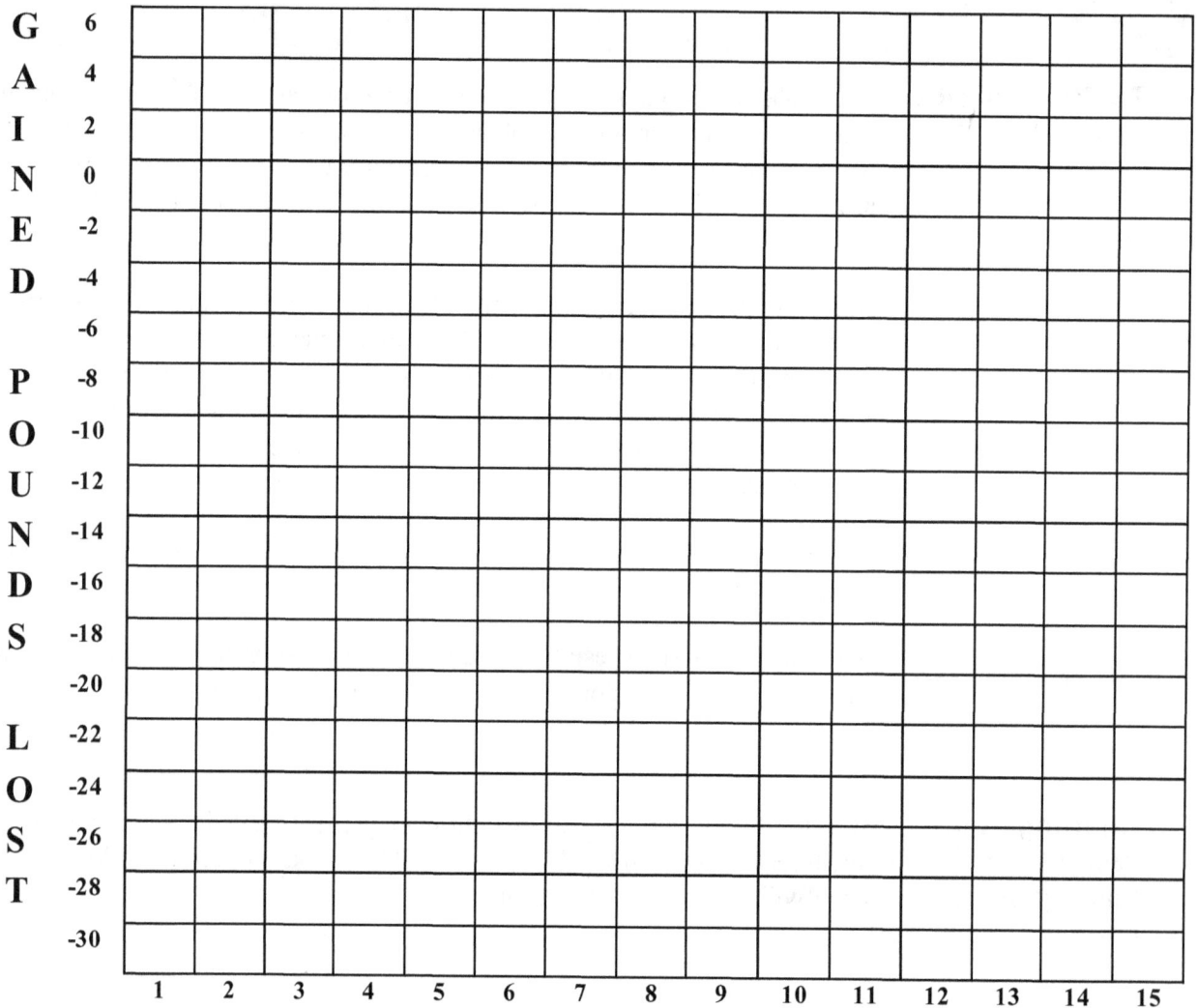

| | | 1 | 2 | 3 | 4 | 5 | 6 | 7 | 8 | 9 | 10 | 11 | 12 | 13 | 14 | 15 |
|---|---|---|---|---|---|---|---|---|---|---|---|---|---|---|---|---|
| **G** | 6 | | | | | | | | | | | | | | | |
| **A** | 4 | | | | | | | | | | | | | | | |
| **I** | 2 | | | | | | | | | | | | | | | |
| **N** | 0 | | | | | | | | | | | | | | | |
| **E** | -2 | | | | | | | | | | | | | | | |
| **D** | -4 | | | | | | | | | | | | | | | |
| | -6 | | | | | | | | | | | | | | | |
| **P** | -8 | | | | | | | | | | | | | | | |
| **O** | -10 | | | | | | | | | | | | | | | |
| **U** | -12 | | | | | | | | | | | | | | | |
| **N** | -14 | | | | | | | | | | | | | | | |
| **D** | -16 | | | | | | | | | | | | | | | |
| **S** | -18 | | | | | | | | | | | | | | | |
| | -20 | | | | | | | | | | | | | | | |
| **L** | -22 | | | | | | | | | | | | | | | |
| **O** | -24 | | | | | | | | | | | | | | | |
| **S** | -26 | | | | | | | | | | | | | | | |
| **T** | -28 | | | | | | | | | | | | | | | |
| | -30 | | | | | | | | | | | | | | | |

**WEEK**

# Chapter 4

# MONITORING CALORIC AND NUTRITIONAL INTAKE

## Overview

Nutrition is the process by which your body consumes food and uses it for growth, tissue replacement and sustenance. The study of nutrition is based on concepts and principles that have been established and tested by scientific method. Poor nutritional status can have a profound effect on physical and mental capabilities and affects all functions of the human body. All living organisms need good nutrition to grow and function properly.

**Food Nutrients**     There are six nutrients essential for human growth and sustenance.

## Table 4-1.  The Essential Food Nutrients

| **Carbohydrates** |
|:---:|
| **Proteins** |
| **Fats** |
| **Vitamins** |
| **Minerals** |
| **Water** |

**Calories**     Carbohydrates, proteins, and fats provide the body with **calories**. A calorie is a unit of fuel the body can convert to energy. *Vitamins, minerals, and water provide no calories.* Table 4-2 shows the caloric value based on weight for each nutrient.

**Calories**

## Table 4-2. Caloric Value of Nutrients

| *Nutrient* | *Caloric Value* |
|------------|-----------------|
| **Carbohydrate:** | *4* Calories per gram |
| **Protein:** | *4* Calories per gram |
| **Fat:** | *9* Calories per gram |
| **Alcohol\*** | *7* Calories per gram |

*\* Alcohol contains calories but has no nutritional value.*

**Importance of Fluids**

Although water consumption is not included on your food records, this does not mean it isn't important. Water does not contain calories, however, it is essential to maintain good health. In fact without water, death occurs within days. Your body is approximately 40-60% water. Water is essential for the process of digestion and absorption of nutrients, and excretion of metabolic wastes. Water plays a direct role in the regulation of body temperature, which becomes especially important with physical activity in warm weather.

There is nothing "magical" with regards to weight loss and drinking water Water will not "flush" fat out of your body, but it will keep you well hydrated and aid in the elimation of toxins from your body. Some people report that increasing their water intake keeps them from overeating, especially at mealtime. Water is supplied from both food and liquids. Foods, mainly fruits and vegetables, contain water. There is no provision for water storage in the body; therefore, the amount lost every 24 hours must be replaced to maintain health. *Normally, about 64 ounces of water (eight 8-ounce cups) are required each day by a sedentary adult living in a normal environment.*

**Guidelines for a Balanced Diet**

For optimal health, a person should consume nutrients in a balanced manner. The American Heart Association and the American Dietetic Association have established a healthy daily balance of carbohydrates, proteins, and fats.

**Guidelines for a Balanced Diet**

# Table 4-3. Recommended Daily Caloric Balance

| Nutrient | Daily Amount |
|----------|--------------|
| Carbohydrate: | 55-60% |
| Protein: | 12-15% |
| Fat: | 30% or less |
|    Polyunsaturated | 10% " |
|    Monounsaturated | 10% " |
|    Saturated | 10% " |

*Source:* Food & Nutrition Guide, *American Heart Association (1996)*

**Types of Fats**

The major kinds of fats in the foods we eat are **saturated, polyunsaturated, monounsaturated** and *trans* **fatty acids. Saturated fats,** *trans* **fats and dietary cholesterol raise blood cholesterol. A high level of cholesterol in the blood is a major risk factor for coronary heart disease, which leads to heart attack.**

Limit foods high in saturated fat, *trans* fat and/or cholesterol, such as full-fat milk products, fatty meats, tropical oils, partially hydrogenated (HI'dro-jen-a-tid or hi-DROJ'en-a-tid) vegetable oils and egg yolks.

Saturated fat and *trans* fat intake should not exceed 10 percent of total calories each day for healthy people. Total fat intake (saturated, trans, monounsaturated, polyunsaturated) should be less than 30 percent of total calories.

**Saturated Fatty Acids**

Saturated fatty acids have all the hydrogen the carbon atoms can hold. Saturated fats are usually solid at room temperature, and they're more stable -- that is, they don't combine readily with oxygen. **Saturated fats and** *trans* **fats are the main dietary factors in raising blood cholesterol** The main sources of saturated fat in the typical American diet are foods from animals and some plants.

**Trans Fat**

*Trans* fats are unsaturated, but they can raise total and LDL ("bad") cholesterol and lower HDL ("good") cholesterol. *Trans* fats result from adding hydrogen to vegetable oils used in commercial baked goods and for cooking in most restaurants and fast-food chains.

**Hydrogenated Fats**

During food processing, fats may undergo a chemical process called hydrogenation (hi"dro-jen-A'shun or hi-DROJ'en-a"shun). Hydrogenate means to add hydrogen, or, in the case of fatty acids, to saturate. The process changes liquid oil, naturally high in unsaturated fatty acids, to a more solid and more saturated form. The greater the degree of

**Hydrogenated Fats (cont.)**

hydrogenation, the more saturated the fat becomes. Many commercial products contain hydrogenated or partially hydrogenated vegetable oils.

Recent studies suggest that these fats may raise blood cholesterol. **Hydrogenated fats in margarine and other fats are acceptable if the product contains liquid vegetable oil as the first ingredient and no more than 2 grams of saturated fat per tablespoon.** The fatty acid content of most margarines and spreads is printed on the package or label. Liquid and soft tub margarines contain little saturated fat or *trans* fat.

**Polyunsaturated/ Monounsaturated Fats**

Polyunsaturated and monounsaturated fatty acids are two types of unsaturated fatty acids. Unsaturated fats have at least one unsaturated bond -- that is, at least one place that hydrogen can be added to the molecule. They're often found in liquid oils of vegetable origin.

Polyunsaturated oils are liquid at room temperature and in the refrigerator. They easily combine with oxygen in the air to become rancid. Common sources of polyunsaturated fats are listed in the table below.

Monounsaturated oils are liquid at room temperature but start to solidify at refrigerator temperatures. See the table below for sources.

## Table 4-4.  Sources of Fat

| Type of Fat | Source |
| --- | --- |
| Polyunsaturated fats | safflower, sesame, soy, corn and sunflower-seed oils, nuts and seeds |
| Monounsaturated fats | olive, canola and peanut oils, avocados |

**What Constitutes a Low Fat Diet?**

A low-fat diet is approximately 60-65 grams of fat for men and 50 grams of fat for women. A rule of thumb recommended by dietitians is to select entrees that contain *less than 15 grams of fat*. Vegetables and side dishes should be prepared without added margarine, cheese, or rich sauces. Salads and desserts should total 5 grams of fat or less. Beverages should be calorie-free water or unsweetened iced tea.

## Table 4-5. Sample Low Fat Distribution by Meals

|  | Men | Women |
|---|---|---|
| Breakfast | 10 grams | 10 grams |
| Lunch | 25 | 20 |
| Dinner | 25 | 20 |
| *Total* | *60 grams* | *50 grams* |

**Fat Calories and Weight Loss**

Are fat calories worse for the weight watcher than carbohydrate and protein calories? The answer is yes. The body metabolizes dietary fat differently than it processes carbohydrate and protein. Dietary fat (fat found in our food) is very similar in composition to body fat, so it takes less energy to convert dietary fat to body fat (remember, 1 gram carbohydrate = 4 calories and 1 gram fat = 9 calories). Not only is it healthier to eat less fat, it is also a better way to control your weight. An important point to remember is:

> **All calories consumed in excess of daily needs are converted to fat.**

**Fat Calories and Weight Loss**

## Table 4-6. The Caloric Density of Fat

> **One Pound FAT TISSUE = 3500 Calories**

**Energy Balance Equation**

*Energy Balance* = the difference between the number of calories you eat (*Intake*) and the number of calories you burn (*Output*). To **lose** weight, you need to have a *calorie deficit*, which means you burn more calories than you take in. On the other hand, when you consume more calories than you burn, you gain weight. Table 4-7 illustrates this equation.

## Table 4-7. Energy Balance Equation

| | |
|---|---|
| **Energy Balance:** | Intake = Output |
| **Energy Gain:** | Intake is greater than Output |
| **Energy Loss:** | Output is greater than Intake |

## Determining Daily Caloric Need

Now let's determine your calorie needs in a day. *You already completed the first step back in Chapter 2 when you determined your target body weight.*

*Note: This is not the weight you need to obtain for Coast Guard height/weight standards. The Coast Guard's height/weight standards represents the maximum allowable weight allowed for your height, frame size, and gender. They are from a policy standpoint and not necessarily the healthiest weight. As a general rule of thumb, the Coast Guard maximum allowable weight standards are higher than what would be considered your target healthy weight.*

**Estimating Energy Needs**

Energy needs are based on daily output or expenditures expressed in calories. The major contributors to energy expenditure are:

- **Basal Metabolic Rate (BMR)** - this is the energy needed to maintain life.

- **Digestion** - a small amount of energy is needed to digest food. This is calculated in the BMR equation.

- **Physical Activity** - energy is needed during physical activity. Estimate your physical activity factor from Worksheet 4-1.

Your total daily estimated energy requirement is the amount of calories you need to offset the energy expended through your BMR and physical activity and to maintain an energy balance of zero. *Calculate your daily energy needs in Worksheets 4-1 & 4-4.*

**Figuring Daily Caloric Needs**

## Worksheet 4-1. Figuring Your Daily Calorie Needs

### Step 1. Determine Your BMR.

| Gender | Age | Age Factor x Body Wt. + Variable |
|--------|-----|----------------------------------|
| Men | 18-30 | 6.95 x Body Weight (lbs.) + 679 |
| | 30-60 | 5.27 x Body Weight (lbs.) + 879 |
| Women | 18-30 | 5.77 x Body Weight (lbs.) + 496 |
| | 30-60 | 3.95 x Body Weight (lbs.) + 829 |

BMR = _____ x _____ + _____

            Age Factor        Lbs.         Variable

Your BMR is _____ Cal/day

## Worksheet 4-1. Figuring Your Daily Calorie Needs (cont.)

### *Step 2. Determine Your Activity Factor.*

Select your *Activity Factor* after you have determined your BMR. Use Table 4-8 as a guideline to figure this.

## Table 4-8. Physical Activity Factors

**Sedentary (1.2).** Seated and standing activities such as driving, lab work, writing, sitting at a desk, typing, cooking, playing cards or a musical instrument.

**Moderately Active (1.3).** Sedentary activities PLUS walking on a level surface, house cleaning, child care, carpentry, restaurant work, gardening, carrying a heavy load, sports & fitness activities with low fitness ratings such as bowling, golf, sailing, baseball, volleyball.

**Very Active (1.4).** Moderate activities PLUS heavy manual labor, walking with a load uphill, sports and physical activities with high fitness ratings such as aerobic classes, cross-country skiing, running, weight lifting.

### *Step 3. Determine Your Daily Calorie Needs.*

Daily Calorie Needs = BMR x Activity Factor

*Calorie Needs* = _____ x _____

                      *BMR*                   *Activity Factor*

> *Your Daily Calorie Need is _____ Calories*

*Now, go to page 1-2 and complete Step 5a. on Worksheet 1-1, My Weight Management Plan.*

# Table 4-8. Physical Activity Factors (cont.)

**Determine Daily Fat Calories**

*Step 4. Determine Your Daily Fat Calories.*

After determining calories, we can go one step further and figure your *maximum daily fat intake* in calories and grams.

Maximum Daily Fat Calories = Daily Calorie Needs x 30%

*Maximum Fat* = _____ x _____

                      *Daily Calorie Needs*     *.3 (30%)*

> ### *Your Maximum Daily Fat is* _____ *Fat calories*

**Determine Daily Fat Grams**

*Step 5. Translate Calories into a Daily Fat Budget.*

Daily Fat Budget = Fat Calories divided by 9

*Daily Fat Budget* = _____ divided by 9

                 *Fat Calories*

> ### *Your Daily Fat Budget is* _____ *grams.*

**Adjusting Daily Fat Budget**

Notice that the percent of calories from fat is based on 30%. There is no "rule" that fat calories need to be any less than 30 percent to lose weight, but many people choose to keep fat grams around 20-25 percent of total calories. For some individuals, keeping fat grams less than 20 percent may be unrealistic, possibly unhealthy, and is not recommended.

Worksheet 4-2 will help you determine a fat budget for different percentages of your total daily calories.

# Worksheet 4-2. Adjusting Your Daily Fat Budget

| Your Daily Calorie Intake | Extremely Low Fat 20% | Low Fat 25% | Recommended Fat Intake 30% |
|---|---|---|---|
| 1,200 | 27 | 33 | 40 |
| 1,400 | 31 | 39 | 47 |
| 1,600 | 36 | 44 | 53 |
| 1,800 | 40 | 50 | 60 |
| 2,000 | 44 | 56 | 67 |
| 2,200 | 49 | 61 | 73 |
| 2,400 | 53 | 67 | 80 |
| 2,600 | 58 | 72 | 87 |
| 2,800 | 62 | 77 | 93 |
| 3,000 | 67 | 83 | 100 |
| 3,200 | 71 | 89 | 107 |

*Your Adjusted Daily Fat Budget =* _____ *grams*

*Now, go to page 1-2 and complete Step 5b. on Worksheet 1-1, My Weight Management Plan.*

**Food Guide Pyramid**

One way to keep track of your calories is to write down what you eat and simply tally calories up at the end of the day. This tends to become a time consuming effort, especially if you are not sure of calorie content of food. Also, this does not ensure that you will get a healthy distribution of nutrients. Some people may find this method too confusing or tedious. If this sounds like you, you may want to try using the **food guide pyramid** to plan your meals. This incorporates the concept of servings (portion control), but is more visual and emphasizes what foods to increase in your diet and what foods to limit.

# Table 4-9. The Food Guide Pyramid

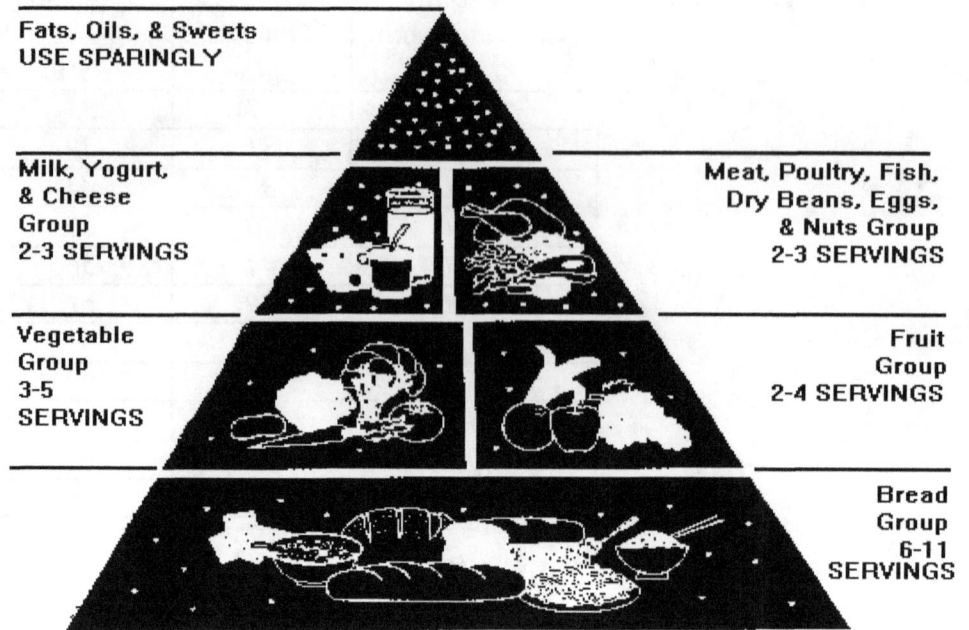

Fats, Oils, & Sweets
USE SPARINGLY

Milk, Yogurt,
& Cheese
Group
2-3 SERVINGS

Meat, Poultry, Fish,
Dry Beans, Eggs,
& Nuts Group
2-3 SERVINGS

Vegetable
Group
3-5
SERVINGS

Fruit
Group
2-4 SERVINGS

Bread
Group
6-11
SERVINGS

**How to Measure Food Portions**

Measuring is essential for portion control. For instance, some people eat the right foods, they just eat too much. Most of us just place food on our plates without realizing how much we actually eat. Measuring cups, spoons, and a plastic kitchen scale are recommended. Starches and milk are measured with measuring cups, whereas meat is weighed on a scale (after cooking).

**How to Measure
Food Portions**

<u>**Table 4-10. What Counts as a Serving?**</u>

**Breads, Cereals, Rice, and Pasta**

1 slice of bread, 1/2 bagel, 1 tortilla, 1/2 pita pocket bread
$^1/_2$ cup of cooked rice, pasta, barley, grits, etc.
$^1/_2$ cup of cooked cereal
1 ounce of ready-to-eat cereal
2/3 cup pretzels

**Vegetables**

$^1/_2$ cup of chopped raw or cooked vegetable
1 cup of leafy raw vegetable

**Fruits**

1 average piece of fruit or melon wedge
$^3/_4$ cup of juice (6 oz.)
$^1/_2$ cup of canned fruit, applesauce, cranberry sauce
$^1/_4$ cup of dried fruit

**Milk, Yogurt, and Cheese**

1 cup of milk or yogurt (8 oz.)
$1^1/_2$ - 2 ounces of cheese (about 2 slices)
1/2 cup cottage or ricotta cheese, ice cream

**Meat, Poultry, Fish, Dry Beans, Eggs, and Nuts**

$2^1/_2$ - 3 ounces of cooked lean meat, poultry, fish
$^1/_2$ cup of cooked beans
1 egg
2 tablespoon of peanut butter
1/4 cup of nuts

**Fats, Oils, and Sweets**

1 tablespoon
*Use sparingly*

**How to Measure Food Portions**

Table 4-11. Visual Guides for Measuring Servings

**1 cup = 1 fist**

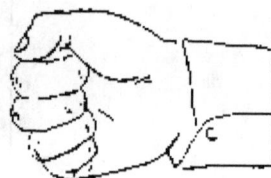

**3 ounces meat, poultry, or fish = woman's palm**

**Or a deck of cards**

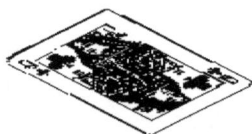

**1 Ounce = 1 Thumb**

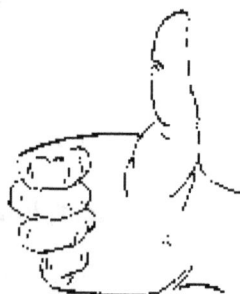

**1 Teaspoon = 1 Thumb Tip**

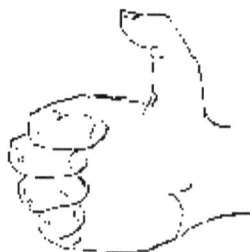

## Table 4-12.  Suggested Food Pyramid Servings

| Total calories | Bread group | Veg. group | Fruit group | Milk group | Meat group | Fat grams |
|---|---|---|---|---|---|---|
| 1200 | 4 | 3 | 2 | 2 | 2 | 35 |
| 1400 | 5 | 3 | 2 | 2 | 2 | 40 |
| 1600 | 6 | 3 | 2 | 2-3 | 2 | 45 |
| 1800 | 8 | 4 | 3 | 2 | 2 | 50 |
| 2000 | 9 | 4 | 3 | 2-3 | 2 | 55 |
| 2200 | 11 | 5 | 4 | 2-3 | 3 | 60 |
| 2400 | 12 | 5 | 5 | 2- 3 | 3 | 65 |
| 2800 | 12 | 6 | 5 | 3 | 3 | 75 |

As you can see, the food guide pyramid is a method of using serving sizes
(portions) as a substitute for calorie counting.  It also helps you achieve a
balanced diet based on the nutritional balance 25-30% Fats, 55-60%
Carbohydrates, 10-15% Protein.  Ideally, calories should be spread out
evenly throughout the day.  You may choose to eat 3, 4, 5, or 6 times per
day.  There is no one best way; it's an individual preference.  Consider
your lifestyle, work schedule, and family priorities, and decide what works
best for you.  Foods are not judged as being "better" or "bad" for you, and
no foods are prohibited! What is important is to examine how much food
you eat and how often.

## Planning Meals According to the Food Pyramid

You may choose to distribute calories for the day as you see fit. However,
*weight loss efforts are enhanced when breakfast is not skipped.* Ideally,
more calories are consumed earlier in the day when energy for activity is
needed, which would make breakfast and lunch the biggest meals of the
day. The following guideline can be used in combination with Table 4-12,
*Suggested Food Servings Guide.*

<u>**Table 4-13. Sample Food Pyramid Meal Planning**</u>

### 1200 Calorie Meal Plan

| | | |
|---|---|---|
| 40 gm. Fat | | Less than 3000 mg sodium |
| 45 gm. Protein | | Less than 300 mg cholesterol |
| 165 gm. Carbohydrate | | |
| Breakfast | 250 Calories | |
| Lunch | 500 Calories | |
| Dinner | 350 Calories | |
| Snacks | 100 Calories | |

### 1400 Calorie Meal Plan

| | | |
|---|---|---|
| 45 gm. Fat | | Less than 3000 mg sodium |
| 55 gm. Protein | | Less than 300 mg cholesterol |
| 190 gm. Carbohydrate | | |
| Breakfast | 300 Calories | |
| Lunch | 600 Calories | |
| Dinner | 400 Calories | |

### 1600 Calorie Meal Plan

| | | |
|---|---|---|
| 50 gm. Fat | | Less than 3000 mg sodium |
| 60 gm. Protein | | Less than 300 mg cholesterol |
| 220 gm. Carbohydrate | | |
| Breakfast | 350 Calories | |
| Lunch | 650 Calories | |
| Dinner | 450 Calories | |
| Snacks | 150 Calories | |

# Table 4-13.  Sample Food Pyramid Meal Planning (cont.)

**Sample Meal Plans (cont.)**

## 1800 Calorie Meal Plan

| | | |
|---|---|---|
| 60 gm. Fat | | Less than 3000 mg sodium |
| 65 gm. Protein | | Less than 300 mg cholesterol |
| 250 gm. Carbohydrate | | |
| Breakfast | 400 Calories | |
| Lunch | 700 Calories | |
| Dinner | 500 Calories | |
| Snacks | 200 Calories | |

## 2000 Calorie Meal Plan

| | | |
|---|---|---|
| 65gm. Fat | | Less than 3000 mg sodium |
| 75 gm. Protein | | Less than 300 mg cholesterol |
| 275 gm. Carbohydrate | | |
| Breakfast | 500 Calories | |
| Lunch | 750 Calories | |
| Dinner | 550 Calories | |
| Snacks | 200 Calories | |

## 2200 Calorie Meal Plan

| | | |
|---|---|---|
| 70gm. Fat | | Less than 3000 mg sodium |
| 85 gm. Protein | | Less than 300 mg cholesterol |
| 300 gm. Carbohydrate | | |
| Breakfast | 550 Calories | |
| Lunch | 835 Calories | |
| Dinner | 615 Calories | |
| Snacks | 220 Calories | |

## Table 4-13. Sample Food Pyramid Meal Planning (cont.)

**Sample Meal Plans (cont.)**

### 2400 Calorie Meal Plan

80 gm. Fat                    Less than 3000 mg sodium

90 gm. Protein                Less than 300 mg cholesterol

330 gm. Carbohydrate *(complex rather than simple)*

| | |
|---|---|
| Breakfast | 600 Calories |
| Lunch | 910 Calories |
| Dinner | 670 Calories |
| Snacks | 240 Calories |

### 2800 Calorie Meal Plan

90 gm. Fat                    Less than 3000 mg sodium

105 gm. Protein               Less than 300 mg cholesterol

385 gm. Carbohydrate *(complex rather than simple)*

| | |
|---|---|
| Breakfast | 700 Calories |
| Lunch | 1065 Calories |
| Dinner | 785 Calories |
| Snacks | 280 Calories |

Make gradual changes in your selection of foods and cooking methods. Healthy eating requires making smart food selections throughout your life. Choosing a food that is lower in nutrition or higher in calories occasionally does not mean your overall diet is bad -- just make those foods the exception in your diet, not the rule.

## Table 4-14.  Sample Low-fat Food Substitutes And Cooking Methods

**Additional Suggestions are found in Appendix B**

| *Try:* | *In Place of:* |
|---|---|
| ***Grains*** | |
| Whole grains & pastas, brown rice | Bleached, white or processed variety |
| Cooking pastas & rice in broth | Cooking pastas & rice with butter or oil |
| ***Vegetables/Fruits*** | |
| Low/non fat salad dressings or vinaigrettes | Creamy salad dressings |
| Vegetables marinated in herbs, lemon or lime juice | Adding butter to vegetables |
| ***Meats*** | |
| Ground turkey, extra-lean beef, trimmed red meats | Ground beef |
| Canadian bacon or ham | Bacon |
| 2 egg whites | 1 whole egg |
| Poultry or fish | Marbled red meats |
| Steaming, broiling, baking, grilling | Frying |
| ***Dairy*** | |
| Non-fat sour cream, yogurt, cottage cheese | Sour cream |
| Skim or 1% milk | Whole milk or nondairy creamer |
| Low-fat cottage cheese | Cheese |
| ***Fats*** | |
| Applesauce for baking | Oil |
| Wine or broth-based sauces | Cream, butter, and oil sauces |
| Canola, olive or safflower oils | Animal fats, coconut or peanut oils |
| Cocoa | Chocolate |
| Spray butter or margarine | Butter |

# Table 4-15.  Fat Content of Selected Food Pyramid Items

This table shows how to identify low-fat foods according to the food groups on the Food Pyramid. Make choices and substitutions from the left hand columns.

**Fat Content of Selected Foods**

| | 0-10% | 10-30% | 30-50% | 50-75% | 75-100% |
|---|---|---|---|---|---|
| *Breads, cereals, rice, pasta* | Many dry cereals and breads, rice, pasta, tortillas, pretzels | Plain popcorn, hot cereals, some breads | Granola, popcorn w/butter, crackers, biscuit, muffin | croissant | |
| *Vegetables and fruits* | Most fresh, frozen, canned, and dried fruits and vegetables | | French fries, onion rings | Potato chips, coconut | Avocados, olives |
| *Milk, yogurt, and cheese* | Nonfat milk, yogurt, and cottage cheese | Low-fat cottage cheese and yogurt, 1% & 2% milk, buttermilk | Whole milk, regular ice cream | Most cheeses, rich ice cream | Half & half, cream cheese, sour cream, heavy cream |
| *Meat, poultry, fish, dry beans, eggs, nuts* | Skinless turkey breast, haddock, cod, most dry beans, egg whites | Skinless white chicken meat, halibut, shrimp, clams, tuna in water, red snapper, trout, low-fat tofu | Beef top round, broiled steak, ham, skinless dark poultry meat, salmon, mackerel, swordfish | Roast beef, ground chuck, pork, lamb, veal chops, poultry with skin, tuna in oil, regular tofu, eggs | Salami, bacon, hot dogs, spare ribs, most nuts and seeds, peanut butter, egg yolks |
| *Combination Foods* | Clear soup (bouillon) | Most broth-based soups, vegetarian chili | Hamburger, lasagna, chili with meat, potato salad, vegetable and cheese pizza, macaroni & cheese, enchiladas | Cheeseburger, meat pizza, large, meat, poultry or cheese sandwich, taco salad | |
| *Fats, oils and sweets* | Hard candy, chewing gum | | | Chocolate bar | Butter, margarine, vegetable oil, mayonnaise, salad dressing |

*Source:* Fit and Well, *Fahey, Insel and Roth (Mayfield Publishing, 1999)*

**Food Portion Sizes**

# Worksheet 4-3. Food Pyramid Portion Size Quiz

*The following quiz will help you review your understanding of food portion sizes*

1.  An ounce and a half of hard cheese- one serving from the dairy group- looks like
    a.  one domino
    b.  two dominoes
    c.  three dominoes

2.  A half cup of cooked pasta-a serving from the grain group- most easily fits into
    a.  an ice cream scoop (the kind with a release handle)
    b.  one coffee cup
    c.  two coffee cups

3.  One drink of wine roughly fills
    a.  two-thirds of a coffee cup
    b.  one coffee cup
    c.  two coffee cups

4.  One serving of green grapes consists of how many grapes?
    a.  10
    b.  15
    c.  20

5.  Three ounces of beef, a serving's worth, most closely resembles
    a.  a *TV Guide*
    b.  a regular bar of soap
    d.  a small bar of soap (as from a hotel)

6.  One serving of Brussels sprouts consists of how many sprouts?
    a.  4
    b.  8
    c.  12

7.  Two tablespoons of olive oil more or less fill
    a.  a shot glass
    b.  a thimble
    c.  a Dixie cup

8.  Two tablespoons of peanut butter make a ball the size of
    a.  a marble
    b.  a tennis ball
    c.  a Ping-Pong ball

9.  How many shakes of a five-hole salt shaker does it take to reach one teaspoon- the maximum RDA?
    a.  5
    b.  10
    c.  60

10. In a pound cake or coffee cake loaf, a serving is the width of
    a.  one finger
    b.  two fingers
    c.  four fingers

**Answers:** 1. C; 2. A; 3. A; 4. A; 5. B; 6. A; 7. A; 8. C; 9. C; 10. A

# The Food Pyramid Record

A Food Pyramid Record is a good way to establish a rough idea of your current eating habits, and determining what and how much you eat. The Record is based on the Food Pyramid guidelines.

**Instructions for Keeping a Food Pyramid Record**

1. Record for two days during the week and one weekend day.

2. Choose days that are typical of your food intake.

3. Use a new page for each day.

4. Record each meal/snack/beverage immediately after you eat it (it is hard to remember at the end of the day).

5. Record each food item on a separate line.

6. If additional space is required for the same day, continue on the back or use an extra form.

7. Write down every bit of food and beverage that goes into your mouth -- even snacks (i.e. gum, hard candy).

8. Be accurate with your portion sizes (this will become easier with practice).

9. List each separate ingredient for mixed dishes (sandwiches, casseroles, salads, etc.) on a separate line fully describe everything you eat and drink in detail (e.g. "chicken thigh, skin not eaten", "low-calorie French Dressing", "whole milk", "regular coffee with creamer", etc.)

10. Be sure you are clear about what constitutes a food portion. Use the enclosed guides.

# Worksheet 4-4. Food Pyramid Record -- Weekday #1

Date _____

| FOOD DESCRIPTION | AMOUNT | B-C-R-P | V | F | M , P , F | M , Y , C | F, O, S |
|---|---|---|---|---|---|---|---|
| | | | | | | | |
| | | | | | | | |
| | | | | | | | |
| | | | | | | | |
| | | | | | | | |
| | | | | | | | |
| | | | | | | | |
| | | | | | | | |
| | | | | | | | |
| | | | | | | | |
| | | | | | | | |
| | | | | | | | |
| | | | | | | | |
| | | | | | | | |
| | | | | | | | |
| | | | | | | | |
| | | | | | | | |
| | | | | | | | |
| | | | | | | | |
| | | | | | | | |
| | | | | | | | |

B-C-R-P = Bread, Cereals, Rice, Pasta; V= Vegetables; F= Fruits; M-P-F= Meat, Fish, Poultry; M-Y-C= Milk, Yogurt, Cheese; F-O-S= Fats, Oil, Sweets

4 - 21

**Worksheet 4-4. Food Pyramid Record -- Weekday #2**

Date _____

| FOOD DESCRIPTION | AMOUNT | B-C-R-P | V | F | M , P , F | M,Y,C | F, O, S |
|---|---|---|---|---|---|---|---|
| | | | | | | | |
| | | | | | | | |
| | | | | | | | |
| | | | | | | | |
| | | | | | | | |
| | | | | | | | |
| | | | | | | | |
| | | | | | | | |
| | | | | | | | |
| | | | | | | | |
| | | | | | | | |
| | | | | | | | |
| | | | | | | | |
| | | | | | | | |
| | | | | | | | |
| | | | | | | | |
| | | | | | | | |
| | | | | | | | |
| | | | | | | | |
| | | | | | | | |
| | | | | | | | |

B-C-R-P = Bread, Cereals, Rice, Pasta; V= Vegetables; F= Fruits; M-P-F= Meat, Fish, Poultry; M-Y-C= Milk, Yogurt, Cheese; F-O-S= Fats, Oil, Sweets

4 - 22

# Worksheet 4-5. Food Pyramid Record -- Weekend

Date _____

| FOOD DESCRIPTION | AMOUNT | B-C-R-P | V | F | M , P, F | M, Y, C | F, O, S |
|---|---|---|---|---|---|---|---|
| | | | | | | | |
| | | | | | | | |
| | | | | | | | |
| | | | | | | | |
| | | | | | | | |
| | | | | | | | |
| | | | | | | | |
| | | | | | | | |
| | | | | | | | |
| | | | | | | | |
| | | | | | | | |
| | | | | | | | |
| | | | | | | | |
| | | | | | | | |
| | | | | | | | |
| | | | | | | | |
| | | | | | | | |
| | | | | | | | |
| | | | | | | | |
| | | | | | | | |

B-C-R-P = Bread, Cereals, Rice, Pasta; V= Vegetables; F= Fruits; M-P-F= Meat, Fish, Poultry; M-Y-C= Milk, Yogurt, Cheese; F-O-S= Fats, Oil, Sweets

4 - 23

# Meals: Frequency and What About Skipping?

**Importance of Breakfast**

Don't skip meals, especially breakfast. A common excuse for skipping breakfast is NO TIME. If you are one of those people who are rushed in the morning, PLAN AHEAD! Breakfast does not have to be a big production, but it does require some advance planning, usually the night before. Many people eat something they can pack and carry with them to eat at work. IF YOU HAVE TIME TO DRINK A CUP OF COFFEE, YOU HAVE TIME TO EAT BREAKFAST.

The one pattern you **should not** follow is to skip breakfast, maybe lunch (or maybe not), and have the bulk of your daily calories consumed after 4 p.m. This unhealthy dietary habit is common among Coast Guard members. Research shows that approximately 90% of people with a weight problem skip at least one or two meals daily, with breakfast being the most frequently missed. *Skipping meals affects your body in the following ways:*

1) Metabolism will lower due to the body's survival mechanism sometimes called "anti-starvation" mechanism. Latest research shows a temporary increase in metabolism of up to 50 percent after eating breakfast.

2) People will generally make up for the calories they missed by overeating in the evening.

# Reading Food Labels

**Overview**

In 1990, Congress passed legislation requiring manufacturers to have standardized food labels on all products. The food label was chosen in 1992 and was required to be on all products by May 1993 (some extensions were granted until 1994). The word "standardized" is very important.

Prior to this legislation, many manufacturers used unrealistic portion sizes to make their products look better. Also, there was great confusion among labeling terms such as "light." "Light" could have meant fewer calories to one manufacturer and lighter in color to another. In addition, not all manufacturers chose to label their products. For instance, you would never have seen cookies with a food label before this law. Today, however, it is easy to check the fat and calorie content of what you eat.

Also, the focus of the new food label has changed. Fifty years ago, Americans were concerned with vitamin and mineral deficiencies, as well as malnutrition. Today these deficiencies are extremely rare, and people are dying of lifestyle related diseases (i.e., heart disease, strokes, cancer,

**Food Label
Overview (cont.)**

and diseases related to obesity. For this reason, the new food label focuses on calories, fat, cholesterol, and sodium. Some vitamins and minerals are still listed, but are not as prominent on the new food label.

Despite these changes, the food label is still a bit confusing to some people. Let's discuss the parts of the food label that relate to weight management.

**Food Label
Information**

## Table. 4-16. What Food Label Information Is Most Important for Losing Weight?

**Serving size -**

Is it realistic?

How many portions will I eat?

**Calories-**

How many does 1-serving contain?

Can it fit into the exchange groups?

**Total fat-**

How many fat grams am I eating?

Can I work this into my fat budget?

**% Daily value**

*This is only helpful if your diet is*

*2000 calories per day*

| Nutrition Facts |
| --- |
| Serving Size 1/2 cup (114g) |
| Servings Per Container: 4 |
| Amount Per Serving |

| | | % Daily Value |
| --- | --- | --- |
| Calories 90 | Calories From Fat 30 | |
| *Total Fat 3 g | | 5 % |
| Saturated Fat 0g | | 0 % |
| Cholesterol 0mg | | 0 % |
| Sodium 300mg | | 13 % |
| *Total Carbohydrate 13g | | 4% |
| Dietary Fiber 3g | | 2% |
| *Sugars 3g | | |
| *Protein 3g | | |
| Vitamin A 80% | Vitamin C | 2% |
| Calcium 4% | Iron | 4% |

*Percent Daily Values are based on a 2,000 calorie diet. Your daily values may be higher or lower depending on your calorie needs:

# Nutrient Label Descriptions

**Overview**
When you compare a typical food label to the one in Table 4-15, you will see there are many items we left off. Does this mean they are not important? No, but for the sake of weight management, five items -- *Calories From Fat, Total Carbohydrates, Sugar, Protein*, and *Daily Values* -- are the best to focus on. **Additional food label terms & definitions are found in Appendix C.**

Should you believe everything you read in the product description? What exactly do all those terms mean? The new food labeling laws requires that all terms must be applied uniformly to ensure they mean the same on all products.

**"Calories from Fat"**
This part tells you how many calories are provided by fat (fat grams multiplied by 9 - 9 is the number of calories per gram of fat).

**"Total Carbohydrates"**
Carbohydrates are important nutrients, but for the average weight watcher, counting carbohydrates is not necessary. Most importantly, monitoring total calorie and fat intake is the key for weight control. Monitoring carbohydrates is useful for diabetics and certain athletes (i.e., marathon runners).

**"Sugar"**
Most of us know sugar as "the bad guy," but sugar is a part of total carbohydrates and is not any more fattening than complex carbohydrates. So why is it bad? Sugar (sucrose or table sugar) has no nutritional quality except calories, whereas complex carbohydrates contain fiber and some B vitamins. We call sugar "empty calories." Next time you look at a regular soda can, see how many grams of sugar it contains. Another food to check for sugar is breakfast cereal. All cereal generally has some added sugar. Remember, extra sugar in the cereal means extra calories. Another important point to remember is that sugar is added to low fat products to enhance flavor. Take a moment to compare a regular product to its low fat counterpart.

**"Protein"**
As long as you have a varied diet with adequate servings of dairy products, meat, poultry, fish, beans and legumes, there should be no reason for you to count protein in grams.

**"Daily Values"**
Daily Values are based on a reference diet of 2,000 calories. This would be the approximate calorie intake for *an average male*. Women, the

**"Daily Values"
(cont.)**

elderly, athletes, and very tall, very small, or very active people may need more or less calories. This makes the percent Daily Value of little use to a large number of people. Keep this in mind when evaluating food labels.

## Your Personal Nutrition Assessment

This questionnaire is a tool for your personal use - no one will see it.... So be honest. This involves looking at four key dietary factors.

- **Prudent Nutrition Habits**: general nutritional balance.

- **Calorie Control Habits**: as pertaining to weight loss and gain.

- **Dietary Fat and Cholesterol**: habits that affect cholesterol in the diet.

- **Sodium or Salt Control**: habits that affect blood pressure.

*Following the score sheet is YOUR NUTRITION PLAN, which includes suggestions on how to improve in each category.*

## <u>Worksheet 4-6. Your Personal Nutrition Assessment</u>

*Answer each question according to your usual eating habits. Place the number corresponding to your answer in the space provided to the left of each question.*

**Prudent
Nutrition Habits**

_____ A. How much milk, yogurt, and cheese do you consume in a day?

1. At least 16 ounces of milk or yogurt, or 3 ounces of cheese

2. 8 ounces of milk or yogurt, or 1 ounce of cheese

3. Only use it in cereal or consume it occasionally

4. Do not consume milk, yogurt, or cheese at all

_____ B. How often do you choose to eat potato chips, corn chips, taco chips, olives, nuts, or other similar foods as snacks or with a meal?

1. Very rarely

2. Occasionally

3. Frequently

4. Usually

_____ C. How many times do you eat fruit per day?

1. 4 or more times

2. 2-3 times

3. 1-2 times

4. None

_____ D. How many whole grain breads and cereals, raw fruits and vegetables, and bran products do you eat each day?

1. 4 or more times

2. 2-3 times

3. 1-2 times

4. None

**Prudent Nutrition Habits (cont.)**

_____ E. Which describes your consumption of vegetables?

    1. I snack on raw veggies and eat veggies/salads with most meals

    2. I eat salads and veggies at one meal per day

    3. I only eat veggies 2-3 times per week

    4. I rarely eat veggies

_____ F. How many glasses of water do you drink in one day?

    1. 8 or more glasses

    2. 5-8 glasses

    3. 2-4 glasses

    4. One glass or none

_____ **TOTAL PRUDENT NUTRITION**

**Calorie Control**

_____ A. What most closely describes the amount you eat at one time?

    1. I stop eating when full, even if there is still food on the plate

    2. I select a small amount and clean the plate

    3. I eat what is served and clean the plate

    4. I take second helpings, especially if it tastes good

_____ B. If you wanted to decrease calorie intake, which would you do?

    1. Cut down on meat, sauces, gravy, desserts, and salad dressings

    2. Limit portion sizes

    3. Leave off bread and potatoes

    4. Follow a crash diet for a few days

**Calorie Control
(cont.)**

_____ C. How many alcoholic beverages do you consume?

1.  0-3 drinks per week

2.  1-2 drinks per week

3.  6-10 drinks per week

4.  3-10 drinks at a time, several times per week

_____ D. Do you ever eat until you are so full that you are uncomfortable?

1.  Rarely, or on special occasions

2.  Periodically, 1-2 times per month

3.  Regularly, once a week

4.  Often, every couple of days, or more

_____ E. How many sweets (candy, pastry, cookies, desserts, ice cream, sugar-based beverages) do you eat?

1.  Only on special occasions, or don't eat sweets

2.  1-3 servings per day

3.  4-5 servings per day

4.  6 or more servings per day

_____ F. Which pattern of eating typifies your style?

1.  Regular meals at frequent intervals

2.  Occasionally skipping a meal and/or bingeing

3.  Eating regular for a few days, then bingeing when there is time to relax

4.  Skipping meals during the day and eating all evening

_____ **TOTAL CALORIE CONTROL**

**Fat and
Cholesterol
Control**

\_\_\_\_\_ A. How often do you eat eggs for breakfast or another meal?

1. Less than once per week

2. 2-3 times per week

3. 4-6 times per week

4. 7 or more times per week

\_\_\_\_\_ B. How many times per week do you consume red meat (beef, steak, bacon, lamb, ribs, etc.)?

1. Less than 2 times per week

2. 2-4 times

3. 5-6 times

4. More than 7

\_\_\_\_\_ C. When you prepare or eat poultry (chicken, turkey, Cornish hen), which of the following plans do you most closely follow?

1. Choose white meat, remove the skin and prepare by baking or broiling

2. Choose dark meat, skin removed and bake or broil

3. Bake or broil, skin on and serve with gravy

4. Leave the skin on and fry

\_\_\_\_\_ D. When selecting a salad or sandwich, which of the following "fillings" would you choose from most often?

1. Lentils, kidney beans, peas, pinto or garbanzo beans

2. Turkey, chicken, tuna, lean cuts of meats, peanut butter, low fat cheese

3. Ham, pastrami, hamburger, salami, hot dogs, bacon, hard cheese

4. Same as #3 with cream or hard cheese

**Fat Control (cont.)**

_____ E. When you eat dairy products (milk, yogurt, cheese, ice cream), do you select?

1. Only skim or low-fat products

2. Only light or low-fat products except when selecting ice cream

3. Are not aware of the difference

4. Only enjoy whole fat content dairy products

_____ F. If you were having potatoes, would you choose?

1. Boiled or baked with no added fat

2. Boiled or baked with polyunsaturated margarine/ yogurt

3. Boiled or baked with margarine or butter and sour cream

4. French fries or hash browns

_____ **TOTAL FAT CONTROL**

**Sodium (salt) Control**

_____ A. How frequently do you add salt to your food after it is served at the table?

1. Never

2. Seldom

3. Sometimes

4. Always

_____ B. How many times do you eat at fast food restaurants?

1. Rarely or always selecting a "salad bar" meal

2. Several times per month

3. Once a week

4. Several times per week

**Sodium Control (cont.)**

_____ C. How often do you eat the following foods: hot dogs, bologna, luncheon meat, bacon, ham, sausage?

1. Less than twice per month

2. Several times per month

3. Once or twice a week

4. 3 or more times per week

_____ D. In what form do you most frequently purchase food for meal preparation?

1. Fresh

2. Canned or frozen without salt

3. Canned without sauces

4. Canned, frozen, or dry with sauces and/or seasonings

_____ E. While preparing meals or when eating out, how frequently do you add any or all of the following items to your food: mustard, pickles, relish, soy sauce, ketchup, meat tenderizer, MSG?

1. Less than 3 times per month

2. Several times per week

3. At least once each day

4. More than 3 times per day

_____ F. How often do you use canned soups or dry soup/broth mixes?

1. Less than twice per month

2. Once a week

3. Several times per week

4. Daily

_____ **TOTAL SODIUM (SALT) CONTROL**

_Now transfer your scores from each section to the chart on the next page._

## <u>Worksheet 4-6.  Your Personal Nutrition Assessment (cont.)</u>

| RATING | PRUDENT DIET Score_____ | CALORIE CONTROL Score_____ | FAT CONTROL Score_____ | SODIUM (SALT) Score_____ |
|---|---|---|---|---|
| EXCELLENT | | | | |
| GOOD | | | | |
| FAIR | | | | |
| POOR | | | | |
| VERY POOR | | | | |

**Interpretation**    Scale:  Excellent……………………...….. 6 - 8

Good……………………………...… 9 - 12

Fair …………………………….… 13 - 16

Poor ……………………………….. 17 - 20

Very Poor ………………………… 21 - 24

**Personal
Nutrition Plan**

<u>**Worksheet 4-7. Your Personal Nutrition Plan**</u>

*Improve your score in each nutrition category by incorporating these
strategies into your lifestyle. Selecting three strategies from each of the
lists below will move you one step closer to the EXCELLENT rating. (X)
those you would like to adopt in your behavior.*

**A. Prudent Nutrition Strategies**

_____ Drink 6-8 glasses of water each day

_____ Drink less regular and diet soda, coffee, and tea

_____ Consume at least 2 servings of a low-fat dairy product

_____ Eat more dark green and deep yellow-orange, fruits and
veggies (i. e., spinach, greens, broccoli, carrots, cantaloupe
peaches, yams)

_____ Include a good source of Vitamin C daily (i. e., oranges,
grapefruits, tomatoes, or juices from these fruits)

_____ Select whole grain breads and cereals, including bran
products

_____ Eat raw fruits and veggies whenever possible

**B. Calorie Control Strategies**

_____ Limit intake of sweets, (i. e., candy, cookies, syrup, jelly,
desserts, pastries, donuts, and sweet rolls)

_____ Cut down on alcohol consumption

_____ Refuse second helpings

_____ Take smaller portions

_____ Stop eating when you're full

_____ Cut down on toppings and condiments (sweet and high fat
additions)

_____ Avoid high fat and "junk" foods

# Worksheet 4-7. Your Personal Nutrition Plan (cont.)

**Your Nutrition Plan (cont.)**

## C. Strategies for Reducing Fat Intake

_____ Limit intake of beef and pork to 3 times per week

_____ Eat more fish, skinless poultry and non-meat protein sources

_____ Select low-fat dairy products (skim milk, low fat yogurt, sherbet, frozen yogurt, cottage cheese)

_____ Reduce intake of eggs; use 2 egg whites to equal 1 egg

_____ Avoid toppings and condiments (butter, margarine, cream, sour cream, non-dairy creamer, high fat salad dressing, guacamole, gravy, and sauces)

_____ Avoid fried foods

_____ Choose baked, broiled, boiled, steamed, poached, and marinated foods

_____ Remove visible fat from meat, and skin from poultry

## D. Strategies for Reducing Sodium (salt)

_____ Eliminate salt at the table and avoid salt in cooking

_____ Cut down on use of condiments (i. e., mustard, ketchup, pickles, relish, soy sauce, steak sauce, monosodium glutamate, and meat tenderizers)

_____ Avoid "fast-food" restaurants

_____ Rarely eat convenience foods, (i. e., canned soups, dried soup mixes, TV dinners, boxed and prepared foods)

_____ Avoid processed meats (i. e., hot dogs, sausage, bacon, and luncheon meats)

_____ Substitute raw fruits and veggies for processed snacks and spreads (i. e., chips, nuts, dips, cheese spreads, pretzels, and crackers)

*Now, go to page 1-2 and Complete Step 6 on Worksheet 1-1, My Weight Management Plan.*

# Chapter 5

# MODIFYING Your Eating Patterns

---

**Value of Record Keeping**

Record keeping for food, exercise, moods, stress, etc. is one of the most important lifestyle behaviors you will learn. It is one of the best predictors of weight loss and successful weight maintenance. **People who keep food and exercise records lose more weight and maintain that weight loss compared to people who don't keep records**. Remember that you are looking for patterns of eating. Make photocopies of Worksheet 5-2 and use it daily.

**Assessment of Eating Patterns**

*The Assessment of Eating Patterns* in **Worksheet 5-1** is a simple technique that you can use as an initial step when changing food habits. It involves identifying behavior associated with your food intake. *Awareness is a key step to changing habits.* Subsequent assessments and worksheets in this chapter will help you become clearer about food patterns you wish to modify.

The *Food Record* in **Worksheet 5-2** can be used to document daily behavior associated with your food intake. When beginning to record your daily intake, have it reviewed by someone you feel is a source of support. While your support person may not be an expert in the field of weight loss, talking about issues with food, etc. usually helps identify problem behaviors. Here are some things you may want to look for:

- *How much fat do I really eat?*
- *How many calories do I really eat?*
- *When is my first meal of the day?*
- *Do I skip meals?*
- *Do I eat when I feel anxious, upset or am affected by other moods?*
- *What portion sizes am I consuming?*

> *Most people tend to underestimate their food intake and overestimate their activity level.*

# Worksheet 5-1.  Assessment of Eating Habits

*Answer the following statements as they TYPICALLY apply to you.*

*Yes/No*

| | |
|---|---|
| 1. Have set daily meal times. | |
| 2. Don't eat at the desk or work area. | |
| 3. Take at least 15 minutes per meal. | |
| 4. Don't skip meals. | |
| 5. Don't snack between meals. | |
| 6. Chew food slowly. | |
| 7. Eat home meals only at the dining table. | |
| 8. Don't eat in the kitchen. | |
| 9. Don't do other activities (TV, reading, driving, etc.) while eating. | |
| 10. *Rarely* eat lying down. | |
| 11. Eat about the same amount whether alone or with others. | |
| 12. Stress doesn't affect the amount of food I eat. | |
| 13. Moods don't affect what, when, or how much I eat. | |
| 14. *Rarely* take second helpings. | |
| 15. Feel okay about leaving some food on my plate. | |
| 16. *Rarely* add high-calorie (fats or sugar) condiments, sauces, or dressings- i. e., jam, butter, salad dressing, gravy, mayonnaise, etc. | |
| 17. *Rarely* eat dessert. | |
| 18. Drink 6-8 glasses of fluids daily (excluding coffee, soft drinks, and alcoholic beverages). | |
| 19. Eat fruits and vegetables daily. | |
| 20. *Rarely* eat high-fat fast foods (hamburgers, fries, pizza, tacos, milkshakes, BBQ, etc.) | |

**Interpretation**

A *NO* answer to any of these questions implies a need to modify your eating habits. **Worksheets 5-7 & 5-8** located later in this chapter will assist you in planing changes to your eating habits.

# Worksheet 5-2. Food Record

The Food Record is an effective way to determine associations between the foods you eat and your moods. Keep a complete daily record for stressful days as well as "typical" days. Be sure to record ALL the situations during the day when you ate food or drank beverages.

*Eating Speed:* 1 = slow, 5 = very rapid. *Stress Level:* 1 = not stressed, 5 = very stressed. *Hunger Level:* 1 = not hungry, 5 = starving! Note your mood when you first start eating. Sometimes we don't have the words to describe our moods. Here is a sample list of words that describe emotions: Anxious, calm, happy, nervous, angry, excited, guilty, sad, bored, funny, lighthearted, serious.

| TIME | EATING SPEED (1-5) | PLACE | WITH WHOM | MOOD/ FEELINGS | STRESS LEVEL (1-5) | WHAT WAS EATEN | HUNGER LEVEL (1-5) |
|------|------|------|------|------|------|------|------|
| | | | | | | | |
| | | | | | | | |
| | | | | | | | |
| | | | | | | | |
| | | | | | | | |
| | | | | | | | |
| | | | | | | | |
| | | | | | | | |
| | | | | | | | |
| | | | | | | | |
| | | | | | | | |
| | | | | | | | |
| | | | | | | | |
| | | | | | | | |

**Assessing Compulsive Eating**

# Worksheet 5-3.  Are You a Compulsive Overeater?

*The following assessment will help you determine whether you have control over your eating habits.*

1. _____ Do you eat when you're not hungry?

2. _____ Do you go on binges for no apparent reason?

3. _____ Do you have feelings of guilt and remorse after overeating?

4. _____ Do you give too much time and thought to food?

5. _____ Do you look forward with pleasure and anticipation to the moments when you can eat alone?

6. _____ Do you plan secret eating binges ahead of time?

7. _____ Do you eat sensibly in front of others and later splurge on high fat foods when you're alone?

8. _____ Is your weight affecting the way you live your life?

9. _____ Have you tried to diet for a week - or longer -- only to fall short of your goal?

10. _____ Do you resent the advice of others who tell you to "use a little will power" to stop overeating?

11. _____ Despite evidence to the contrary, have you continued to assert that you can diet "on my own" whenever you wish?

12. _____ Do you crave to eat at a definite time, day or night, other than meal times?

13. _____ Do you eat to escape from worries or troubles?

14. _____ Has your physician ever treated you for overweight?

15. _____ Does your food obsession make you or other unhappy?

**Interpretation**

A *YES* response to three or more of the questions can point to a potential problem with compulsive overeating. You should consider a consultation with the CG Employee Assistance Program (EAP).

*Source: Overeaters Anonymous*

# Worksheet 5-4  Do You Feel Social Pressure to Eat?

**Assessing
Social Pressure**

*This assessment can help you determine how well you cope with social influences on your eating habits. Rate yourself on each of the following statements on how much you agree or disagree with each one.*
*1= Never; 2= Sometimes; 3= Usually; 4= Almost Always; 5= Always.*

*My Score*

| | |
|---|---|
| 1. It's not right to say "no" when someone is just trying to be nice to me. | |
| 2. It's often hard for me to speak up for what I need or want. | |
| 3. I'd rather put my own needs second than hurt someone else's feelings. | |
| 4. It isn't fair to want others to help me in my weight-management efforts. | |
| 5. I shouldn't involve others in my problems. | |
| 6. I need to drink or eat a big entrée at a restaurant in order to make others feel comfortable. | |
| 7. When someone else is paying for it, I feel I may as well take advantage. | |
| 8. Guests who are invited to dinner expect to be treated to fancy (i. e. "high calorie") meals. | |
| 9. A good host or hostess fixes special meals for company, and this involves a "rich" entrée and a sweet dessert. | |
| 10. When invited to dinner, I should show my appreciation by eating well. | |
| 11. Calling ahead to inquire about the menu or making special requests of a hostess is making a nuisance of myself. | |
| 12. Other people depend on me, and their needs come first. | |
| 13. When someone tries to pressure me, I resist, even if what they want me to do is a good idea. | |
| 14. When someone I care about doesn't want me to change, I feel I should do as they ask. | |
| 15. I like the attention and sympathy I get from having a weight problem. | |
| 16. I can't resist food at parties or celebrations. | |
| 17. When I see others eating, I just can't resist getting something to eat too. | |
| 18. It isn't polite to refuse food when someone has prepared it especially for me. | |

**Total Score** _____

**Interpretation**

**18-36:** *Low Pressure Quotient.* Your beliefs are strong enough to help you resist social influences.

**37-53:** *Moderate Pressure Quotient.* Some of your beliefs make it difficult for you to cope with social pressures. Identify which belief keeps you stuck, and change your way of thinking on these.

**54-90:** *High Pressure Quotient.* Much of your belief system makes it harder for you to cope with social influences. You need to challenge your beliefs and make changes about the way you think about them.

# Worksheet 5-5.  What Triggers Your Eating?

*Take this short test and you will understand some of the factors that influence
your eating habit. Score yourself on each statement to what degree the situation
is likely to prompt you start eating. Answer every question.*
*5= Always; 4= Almost Always; 3= Usually; 2= Sometimes; 1= Never*

*My  Score*

| | |
|---|---|
| **A.** Arguing or being in conflict with someone. | |
| **B.** Make excuses to myself about why it's okay to eat. | |
| **C.** Eating is a source of relaxation for me. | |
| **D.** I eat when I feel angry about something. | |
| **E.** When I have run out of my favorite food I find that I'm uncomfortable until I replace it. | |
| **F.** I eat certain foods automatically without being aware of it. | |
| **G.** I eat to stimulate me, to perk myself up. | |
| **H.** Worrying triggers my need for food. | |
| **I.** A strong desire to eat even though I've just eaten or feel "full." | |
| **J.** When I feel uncomfortable or upset about something, I eat. | |
| **K.** Experience fatigue or being over-tired. | |
| **L.** Watching television, reading or doing some other activity while I'm eating. | |
| **M.** Experience trembling, headache, or light-headedness associated with not eating. | |
| **N.** Criticizing myself for being overweight or unable to control my eating. | |
| **O.** I want to eat most when I'm comfortable and relaxed. | |
| **P.** When I feel "blue" or want to take my mind off cares or worries, I eat. | |
| **Q.** I get a real gnawing hunger when I haven't had my favorite food for a while. | |
| **R.** Eat without paying much attention to the amount or the taste of the food. | |
| **S.** Being with others when they are eating, regardless of when I last ate. | |
| **T.** Eat when I experience physical discomfort or pain. | |
| **U.** Feeling inadequate around others. | |

**Scoring**

*Add up your scores for each set of letters:*

A + S + U = _____   B + H + N = _____         C + G + D = _____

D + J + P = _____   E + I + Q = _____         F + L + R = _____

K + T + M = _____

*Transfer the scores to the table on the next page.*

**Influencing Factors**

| FACTOR | YOUR SCORE |
|---|---|
| 1. SOCIAL (A+S+U) | _____ |
| 2. THINKING (B+H+N) | _____ |
| 3. PLEASURE (C+G+0) | _____ |
| 4. EMOTIONAL (D+J+P) | _____ |
| 5. PSYCHOLOGICAL (E+I+Q) | _____ |
| 6. HABIT (F+L+R) | _____ |
| 7. PHYSICAL (K+T+M) | _____ |

**Interpretation**

*Your scores will be between 3 and 15 for each of the factors. Any score above 10 is high.*

The seven factors describe different ways of experiencing and managing feelings, stressors, or situations. *Stimulation* represents the positive feelings people get from eating. Four factors -- *Social, Psychological, Emotional, and Physiological* -- decrease negative feelings by reducing a state of physical discomfort or emotional tension. The sixth factor -- *Thinking/Rationalizing* -- is a pattern of filtering or interpreting events. It influences your emotional or psychological state. The seventh factor -- *Habit*- takes place in the absence of feeling or thinking -- purely an automatic response to a familiar situation.

A score of 11 or more on any factor indicates that this is an important influence on your eating behavior. The higher the score, the more important is your consideration of how it affects your relationship to food.

*In order to make healthy changes in your eating behavior you may have to get along without the gratification and tension reduction food has given you. More important, you will have to find more acceptable and healthier ways of experiencing satisfaction or a reduction in tension or discomfort.* In either case, you need to know just what it is you are getting out of your current eating behavior before you can decide to make healthy changes.

# Understanding the Factors that Trigger Your Eating

**Social**

Interpersonal situations -- work relations, meetings, family, social gatherings, etc. - can be a source for discomfort, tension, conflict, or feelings of inadequacy. If you score high in this factor you may not be handling certain social interactions to your satisfaction. Eating may be your method of reducing the tension or discomfort associated with a particular social situation. Improving your social skills through communication classes, assertiveness and conflict resolution training, or marriage and family counseling can help reduce tension and discomfort in social situations.

**Thinking/ Rationalizing**

Your beliefs and attitudes influence how you feel and react to situations. Beliefs may be developed unconsciously and act as predictors to events. Before an act or a feeling is experienced it exists first as a thought. Attitudes and beliefs form your self-image, sense of competence, ability to handle stressful situations, your relationship to food, etc. Changing the belief can change the feelings and behavior. Positive affirmations and goal setting will help.

**Pleasure/ Stimulation**

It is not always easy to determine whether you use food to feel good, that is to get pleasure, or to keep from feeling bad (Factor #4). Those who do get real stimulation out of eating often find that an honest consideration of the unhealthy effects of their habit is enough to help them modify their use of food. They substitute more appropriate activities that fit the situation-exercise, social events, creative activities, supportive relationships, music, etc.

**Emotional**

Many people use food as a sponge to absorb negative feelings in moments of stress or discomfort, and on occasion it may work. Food is sometimes used as a tranquilizer. When things are going well this kind of food user may find it easy to control their eating, but will be tempted again in times of stress. Again, exercise, relaxation, social outlets, creative activities, etc. may serve as more useful, longer lasting, and healthier substitutes.

**Psychological**

*Craving* or psychological dependence on food is a more intensified development of tension reducing, emotional crutches, or need for pleasure/stimulation. For this person, the preoccupation with food is almost constant. Even when they have just finished eating they are already thinking of the next food they want to eat. Changing eating habits is

| | |
|---|---|
| **Psychological (cont.)** | difficult for this kind of person. For the craving or dependent eater, seeing a physician or a counselor, or enrolling in a structured behavior change program is probably necessary to provide the essential skills or motivation to change. |
| **Habit** | This kind of food user is no longer getting much satisfaction from eating. They just eat without even realizing what they're doing. There is little awareness of the quantity or frequency of eating. For this person, change requires breaking the patterns that have been built up. Keeping a food log is one way to help recognize and break these patterns. Cutting down or reducing the frequency may be effective once there is an increased awareness of the habit. Slowing down and becoming aware of each piece of food is another strategy. |
| **Physical** | Some people have learned to respond to certain physiological conditions - fatigue, pain, muscle tension, headache, etc. - by eating. It is not always easy to determine whether the physical condition is a response to actual hunger. Eating at regularly set times and paying attention to the quantity and quality of the food are key ways of modifying your behavior. In other situations it is important to recognize your "stimulus-response" pattern. In this way the physical "stimulus" (i.e., pain, discomfort) can be used as a trigger to remind you to activate a pre-planned behavior- relaxation, exercise, etc. - rather than the "learned" response. |

## YOUR SELF IMAGE

It is important to create a realistic view of your body. Some people feel bad or have an uncomfortable feeling about their body. This can happen when someone has a picture in their mind of "the perfect body" and tries to achieve it at all costs. Others can only see themselves as fat, even after they have lost a lot of weight. There are useful techniques to develop a more realistic view of yourself. For example, while losing weight, regularly stand unclothed in front of a full-length mirror.

Start taking notice of any changes in your body that have resulted from your weight loss. Or, have someone take a full-length photograph of you (clothed) when you begin your weight-loss program and each month thereafter. Be sure to wear the same clothes each time. Compare the photographs, take note of changes in how you look, and think about how the clothes now feel on you.

# Worksheet 5-6.  Assess Your Body Image

*Using the following scale, score yourself on each statement. Then total your points. 1= Never; 2: Sometimes; 3= Usually; 4= Almost Always; 5= Always*

*My Score*

| | |
|---|---|
| 1. I dislike seeing myself in mirrors. | |
| 2. When I shop for clothing I am more aware of my weight problem and consequently I find shopping for clothes unpleasant. | |
| 3. I'm ashamed to be seen in public. | |
| 4. I Prefer to avoid engaging in sports or public exercise because of my appearance. | |
| 5. I feel embarrassed by my body in the presence of someone of the opposite sex. | |
| 6. I think my body is ugly. | |
| 7. I feel that other people think my body is unattractive. | |
| 8. I feel that my family or friends are embarrassed to be seen with me. | |
| 9. I compare myself with other people to see if they are heavier than I am. | |
| 10. I find it difficult to enjoy non-physical activities involving other people because I'm self-conscious about my appearance. | |
| 11. Feeling guilty about my weight problem preoccupies my thinking. | |
| 12. My thoughts about my body and physical appearance are negative and self-critical. | |

**TOTAL SCORE** _____

**Interpretation**

12-15 Points:  Positive Body Image.

16-24 Points:  Need to develop a healthier body image.

25-60 Points:  Unhealthy body image.

**Food Cues**

You can control environmental cues that contribute to unhealthy eating habits. *Food Cues* are situations that trigger learned or automatic behaviors. For example, replacing candy dishes with fruit bowls can help you cut down on the amount of candy you may eat. Staying away from buffet or cafeteria-style restaurants can reduce the temptation to overeat. Putting your exercise shoes by the front door can remind you to take your daily walks. Complete the following checklist to help control environmental cues.

## Worksheet 5-7. Changing Food Cues

*Using the record below, identify your food cue triggers, describe your typical response to the cue and then develop a new response plan. You can later check your results.*

| Food Cue | Current Response | New Response | Results |
|---|---|---|---|
| Storing Food | | | |
| Eating Methods | | | |
| Serving Food | | | |
| Buying Food | | | |
| Cleaning Up | | | |
| Holidays | | | |
| Weekends | | | |
| After-dinner/evening | | | |
| Where I eat | | | |
| What I do while eating | | | |
| Alcohol | | | |
| Entertaining & parties | | | |
| Eating Out | | | |
| Travel & Vacations | | | |
| Emotions (specify) | | | |
| Stressors (specify) | | | |
| Specific Problem Foods | | | |
| Other Cues (specify) | | | |
| Other Cues (specify) | | | |
| Other Cues (specify) | | | |

***Now, go to page 1-3 and complete Step 7a. on Worksheet 1-1, My Weight Management Plan.***

# Worksheet 5-8. Planning New Eating Behaviors

*The following is a list of positive food behaviors. Check the ones you wish to incorporate into your new food behavior plan.*

_____ Start each day with breakfast.

_____ Eat three regular, planned meals.

_____ Eat meals at scheduled times.

_____ Eliminate between meal snacks.

_____ Choose small, planned snacks.

_____ Plan a menu for each meal.

_____ Don't buy these "problem foods": _____

_____ Practice focused-eating.

_____ Ask for low-cal and/or fat-free substitutes.

_____ Keep problem food out of sight.

_____ Don't sample food during meal preparation.

_____ Don't eat anything after the evening meal.

_____ Measure food portions.

_____ Leave some food on my plate.

_____ Take at least 20 minutes to eat each meal.

_____ Skip seconds.

_____ Use smaller dishes.

_____ Put utensils down between bites.

_____ Let someone else scrape plates.

_____ Sit down while eating.

_____ Don't do anything else while eating.

_____ Share a single serving- especially a high cal dish

# Worksheet 5-8. Planning New Eating Behaviors (cont.)

**Planning New Eating Behaviors (cont.)**

\_\_\_\_\_ Put leftovers away immediately.

\_\_\_\_\_ Don't eat in the car.

\_\_\_\_\_ Don't get snacks for others.

\_\_\_\_\_ Select restaurants with varied menus, including "healthy heart" selections.

\_\_\_\_\_ Avoid the following restaurants/chains: _____.

\_\_\_\_\_ Eat only in "designated eating areas" at home and at work.

\_\_\_\_\_ Low-cal "Snack substitutes" will be: _____.

\_\_\_\_\_ Shop only from a prepared list.

\_\_\_\_\_ Order skim milk or diet soft drinks or low-cal beverages when eating out.

\_\_\_\_\_ Open food packages only when ready to use.

\_\_\_\_\_ Ask others- family, friends, co-workers- not to offer food.

\_\_\_\_\_ Ask someone else to do the grocery shopping.

\_\_\_\_\_ Don't shop when hungry.

\_\_\_\_\_ Cut up fruits & vegetables for snacks.

\_\_\_\_\_ Plan meals the day before or at the beginning of the week.

\_\_\_\_\_ Low-calorie snacks to work.

\_\_\_\_\_ Eat one bite at a time, placing the utensil down between bites.

\_\_\_\_\_ Stay out of the kitchen between meals and after the evening meal.

\_\_\_\_\_ When eating out, share entrees, desserts, sauces, and dressings.

\_\_\_\_\_ When there is an urge to eat, wait at least five minutes.

\_\_\_\_\_ Avoid these trouble spots in the supermarket: _____

\_\_\_\_\_ Other: _____

*Now, go to page 1-3 and complete Step 7b. on Worksheet 1-1, My Weight Management Plan.*

# Chapter 6

# EATING IN COAST GUARD DINING FACILITIES

## Overview

Is it possible to lose weight *and* eat in a Coast Guard dining facility? Yes, and it doesn't mean living on cottage cheese and carrot sticks. This chapter includes the tools needed to eat healthier, as well as empowering you to recommend changes to the Coast Guard dining facilities where you are eating.

**How Are Menus Planned?**

Menus are planned locally by the Food Service Specialist (FS), often using the Armed Forces Menus Standards. Primary considerations for menus are (1) cost, (2) crew preference, (3) balance of the food groups, (4) seasonal availability of foods, (5) cultural difference, and (6) making sure meals contain enough calories and nutrients for a crew - typically, young and hard - working.

**Express Your Needs**

FS personnel want to please the customer. Some ways for service members to request preferences are at point of service. Another option is the suggestion box. Most ships have a menu review board with a representative from each division, and this is an excellent way to provide feedback to the food service division. The chain of command and Command Master Chief are also methods that can be used. Assert your likes and dislikes. Your FS personnel will appreciate the feedback.

Some galleys are more progressive than others, offering and promoting low fat choices. While none are expected to offer "health spa" food, they should be able to provide healthy options, especially if they know their customers are interested.

**Moderate Your Portions**

The Coast Guard is unique from civilian life; that is, the food prepared for you is all-you-can-eat. Going back for seconds or thirds is not unusual. You can have all the low fat selections available, but they are not beneficial if extra helpings are a common occurrence.

**Avoid Second Helpings**

If tempted to continue eating after your first plateful is gone, use your behavior modification strategies. In particular, make your first plateful last at least 20 minutes if possible. Slow down, put your fork down between bites, or sip a non-caloric beverage while eating. Listen to your hunger cues; are you really still hungry or are you craving more food for its flavor or texture? As a last resort, leave the mess hall for another activity if second helpings are too tempting.

**Request Healthy Choices**

## Worksheet 6-1.  Requesting Healthy Galley Menu Choices

*These are some food selections and food preparation methods you can request your Coast Guard dining facility to make available:*

_____Skim milk or 1% milk as the primary milk choice.

_____Entrees or sandwiches that have less that 15 grams of fat per serving.

_____Post which choices fit into a low fat meal plan.

_____Meatless entrees such as spinach lasagna.

_____Meatless entrees such as low fat (low fat cheese) spinach lasagna.

_____Different varieties of baked fish entrees 2-3 times per week.

_____Baked chicken on the speed line.

_____Fresh baked low-fat and low-calorie breads.

_____Fajita bar with low-fat turkey or chicken. Steamed not fried veggies.

_____Side dishes with less than 5 grams of fat.

_____Cooked vegetables without added fat.

_____Potato bar with healthy toppings (non-fat cottage cheese, raw veggies, etc.).

_____Pasta bar with low fat sauces.

_____Fruit toppings such as applesauce or sliced fruit as an alternative to butter or syrup.

_____English muffins and bagels.

_____Low-fat sandwiches such as roast turkey breast with low-fat thousand island on pita bread, whole wheat, or rye.

_____Vegetarian sandwiches.

_____Plain low fat/non fat yogurt.

_____Whole grain cereal, hot cereals and grits without added butter.

_____Position fresh fruit, cereals, yogurt, breads <u>before</u> the grill at breakfast.

_____Leave fat out of vegetables.

_____Label low-fat entrees with red hearts or other identifying marks.

_____Label fat grams on entrees.

_____Fresh fruit.

_____Steamed vegetables.

***Now, go to page 1-3 and complete Step 7c. on Worksheet 1-1, My Weight Management Plan.***

# Worksheet 6-2.  Making Low Calorie Choices at the Galley

*These dining strategies are some common ways you can modify your eating habits for Coast Guard dining facilities. Identify the ones you wish to put into action.*

_____1 percent or skim milk.

_____Sandwiches without processed foods (meat and cheese).

_____Vegetarian sandwiches.

_____Eliminate high calorie condiments - especially mayonnaise, butter, and salad dressing.

_____Raw and cooked vegetables without added fat (sauces and butter).

_____Potato bar with healthy toppings – non fat cottage cheese, raw veggies, etc.

_____Pasta bar without added fat (dressings, cheese sauces, etc.).

_____Meatless entrées such as spinach lasagna.

_____Pass up high calorie, high fat baked sweets- pastries, desserts, cake, donuts, etc.

_____Fajita bar with low-fat turkey or chicken. Steamed not fried veggies.

_____Fruit toppings such as applesauce or sliced fruit as an alternative to butter or syrup.

_____Toasted English muffins or bagels instead of donuts or muffins.

_____Low-fat sandwiches with roast turkey breast, pita bread, whole wheat, rye, and low fat condiments.

_____Non-fat yogurt with fresh fruit.

_____Whole grain cereal, hot cereals and grits (without added butter).

_____Egg substitutes or egg whites only.

_____Skip desserts.

_____Other _____.

***Now, go to page 1-3 and complete Step 7d. on Worksheet 1-1, My Weight Management Plan.***

# Chapter 7

# DINING OUT

## Overview

**What's Included?**

There are many occasions when you find yourself eating away from home. It is likely that you will eat five or more meals per week away from home. *Dining out* includes restaurants, fast-food, special occasions, parties, traveling, vacations, holidays, business trips- basically any occasion when you will be eating away from home and your normal routine. We are often confronted with unusual food choices and are not in complete control of the menu. This is one of the biggest challenges to your eating behavior plan.

Other stressors that affect your eating routine are eating on the run, social pressures and dynamics, new environment, presence of high-calorie food and beverages, alcohol, etc.

**Developing Strategies**

You will need to develop strategies *ahead of time* to manage special occasions. This means being aware of your particular stressor and developing new behaviors to replace typical ones.

## Worksheet 7-1. New Dining Out Behaviors

*After you plan your new dining-out behavior, go to page 1-3 and complete Step 7e on Worksheet 1-1, My Weight Management Plan.*

| Situation or Stressor | Current Behavior | New Food Behavior |
|---|---|---|
| Entertaining - as a host | | |
| Parties - as a guest | | |
| Restaurant dining | | |
| Fast Food restaurants | | |
| Alcoholic Beverages | | |
| Foods & Dishes | | |
| Appetizers | | |
| Salads | | |
| Meats | | |
| Sandwiches | | |
| Vacations | | |
| Business Trips | | |
| Breads | | |
| Pastries | | |
| Desserts | | |
| Fats | | |
| Beverages | | |

# Chapter 8

# MONITORING PHYSICAL ACTIVITY

## Putting Together Your Physical Activity Plan

## "The ultimate cure for obesity is exercise"

*-Covert Bailey, biochemist and well-known lecturer in the study of obesity*

**Overview**

The best exercise plan is *comprehensive* - which includes muscle strength and endurance development, cardiorespiratory, and flexibility exercises. The reality is that your plan may be more restricted due to balancing the factors of personal preference, time, efficiency, calories burned, and equipment availability. However, if you are motivated and make the time a *combined* aerobic and strengthening program makes for successful weight loss. Contact your unit Health Promotion Coordinator or the regional Health Promotion Manager for instruction on the safe and effective use of exercise equipment.

**The FITT Plan**

To create a successful exercise program you must set realistic goals. This is called the *FITT Plan* in which you determine the *Frequency, Intensity, Time*, and *Type* of activity. The worksheets in this chapter will help you develop a personal *FITT* plan.

## Table 8-1. Components of a Complete Exercise Program

1. *Cardioresipratory Exercise (Cardio)*

2. *Muscle Strength and Endurance (MSE)*

3. *Stretching: Warm-up and Cool-down*

**Cardio Activities**

Cardiorespiratory activities are endurance exercises that involve the rhythmic use of large muscles - i.e. the legs and/or arms and shoulders - that is continuous, for an extended period of time, and reflects an increase in heart rate. The word *aerobic* is often used to describe this type of activity. Walking, jogging, swimming, and aerobic dance are some examples of aerobic activity.

**Strength Training**

What exactly is MSE? Muscle strength and endurance, sometimes called weight lifting, resistance training, or strength training, is based on the principle that muscles adapt to the stress or resistance placed upon them. Strength training can significantly increase your progress with fat reduction in one simple yet critical, way: increased muscle = higher resting metabolism!

*Strength training can be accomplished in a few different ways*:

1. Using your body as weight resistance (sit-ups, push-ups).

2. Using weight machines or free weights as resistance.

3. Using resistance tubing.

If strength training is new to you, it is essential to enlist the help of a *trained* person - your unit Health Promotion Coordinator, regional Health Promotion Manager, MWR personnel, local recreation or school personnel, or a certified personal trainer. They can help you determine the most appropriate equipment, how to use equipment safely and effectively, and how to plan a weekly exercise routine. When beginning a strengthening program, proper technique is vital to minimize the risk of injury.

**Stretching**

A warm-up is crucial, as warm muscles are less likely to tear (muscle strain). A warm-up can include a 5-minute jog in place or a brisk walk. Muscles are warmed by increasing the blood flow to them. Stretch *after* warm up - if you begin stretching immediately, muscles are cold and could tear. Stretch slowly and never bounce. Never stretch to the point of pain. A stretch should last 20-45 seconds. A cool-down period is also important, as you want your heart rate to gradually come down to facilitate equal blood distribution to prevent blood pooling and fainting.

## Calorie-burning Goal

**How Much Should I Burn?**

*One pound of fat contains 3500 calories.* If you **reduce** your weekly caloric intake by half that (1750 calories) and **increase** your weekly physical activity to burn the other half (1750 calories) then you are on a realistic, prudent, and safe weight program. The following formula and chart will help you determine the way you can burn those calories. This also helps you set Frequency of exercise - one of the components of your *FITT Plan*.

**Recommended Weekly Goal: Expend 1750 Calories**

## Table 8-2.  Physical Activity Required to Expend 1750 Calories/ Week

4 Days of exercise per week = 435 calories per day

5 Days of exercise per week = 350 calories per day

6 Days of exercise per week = 290 calories per day

7 Days of exercise per week = 250 calories per day

## Table 8-3. Calorie-Burning Formula

*The formula to determine how many calories are burned for a selected activity over a specific period of time:*

**CALORIES  BURNED = Activity X Body Weight X Minutes**

**Calorie Expenditure Chart**

The Worksheet 8-1 (Calorie Expenditure Chart) on the next page will help you figure out how many calories you burn during your exercise session. Select the appropriate activity and intensity level and then calculate based on your body weight and the time you actually spent doing the activity. ***Be sure to subtract rest and stop times.***

**Example**: A 150 lbs. person does moderate walking (4 mph) for 45 minutes (non-stop).

Calories burned = .037 X 150 lbs. X 45 min. = 250 Calories

**Burning Calories**

## <u>Worksheet 8-1. Calculating Calorie Expenditure</u>

| Activity | Cal/Min. | Body Wt. | Time (min.) | Total Calories |
|---|---|---|---|---|
| Aerobics Class (moderate) | .046 | | | |
| Aerobics Class (vigorous) | .062 | | | |
| Basketball (half court) | .045 | | | |
| Basketball (full court) | .071 | | | |
| Cycling (6 mph) | .032 | | | |
| Cycling (8 mph) | .039 | | | |
| Cycling(10mph) | .045 | | | |
| Cycling (13 mph) | .071 | | | |
| Digging | .062 | | | |
| Hiking (moderate) | .051 | | | |
| Hiking (vigorous) | .073 | | | |
| Housecleaning | .029 | | | |
| Jogging (12 min./mi.) | .060 | | | |
| Jogging (10 min./mi.) | .081 | | | |
| Jogging (9 min/mi.) | .088 | | | |
| Painting (a house) | .034 | | | |
| Racquetball(mod. singles) | .049 | | | |
| Racquetball(skilled singles) | .078 | | | |
| Shoveling Snow | .052 | | | |
| Tennis (doubles) | .045 | | | |
| Tennis (skilled singles) | .071 | | | |
| Walking (3 mph) | .026 | | | |
| Walking (4 mph) | .037 | | | |
| Walking (4.5 mph) | .048 | | | |
| Washing the Car | .035 | | | |
| Weight Training- moderate | .058 | | | |
| Weight Training- vigorous | .067 | | | |
| In-line Skating (8 mph) | .041 | | | |
| In-line Skating (12 mph) | .084 | | | |
| In-line Skating (15mph) | .115 | | | |
| Swimming (100 yds@4:00) | .041 | | | |
| Swimming (100 yds@3:00) | .057 | | | |
| Swimming (100 yds@2:00) | .081 | | | |

*Source: Fit and Well (1999)*

# DETERMINING THE APPROPRIATE INTENSITY
# OF PHYSICAL ACTIVITY

There are two easy methods to determine how intense you are exercising.

1.  *Perceived Exertion Scale*

2.  *Target Heart Rate method*

**The Perceived Exertion Scale**

The *Perceived Exertion Scale* is based on studies that show our own subjective estimate of effort (how hard we are exercising) and is highly correlated to actual heart rate, oxygen consumption, and lactic acid produced during exercise. In layman's terms, we should be listening to ourselves during exercise. If the exercise feels too difficult, it probably is. The scale slides with you as you become more physically conditioned. For instance, an out of shape individual may find a 9 min. per mile pace as "very hard," while competitive runner may find the same pace "fairly light." In other words, the scale adapts no matter what shape you are in.

## Table 8-4.  Perceived Exertion Scale

| *How does the exercise feel?* | *Rating* |
|---|---|
| Very, very light | 6-7 |
| Very light | 8-10 |
| Fairly light | 11-12 |
| Somewhat hard | 13-14 |
| Hard | 15-16 |
| Very hard | 17-18 |
| Very, very hard | 19-20 |

**Note**

Your perceived exertion rating X 10 is approximately equal to your heart rate. For example, "Hard" = 15 X 10 or 150 beats per minute. As long as the exercise effort is at the "somewhat hard" to "hard" level, you should be in your target heart rate zone. You'll need to remember to ask yourself periodically during your exercise sessions "how do I feel?"

**Determining Target Heart Rate**

The **Target Heart Rate (THR)** method is commonly used to measure exercise intensity, and relies on checking heart rate (pulse). Exercise should be performed within a specified target heart rate zone. *Target heart rate zone is defined as 65-90 percent of your maximum heart rate.* This will provide the desired effect of aerobic fitness and calorie burning by exercising within this zone. Aerobic fitness is achieved by increased oxygen consumption over time, and heart rate is a convenient indicator of oxygen consumption. The following method is recommended by the American College of Sports Medicine:

### Worksheet 8-2. Calculating Target Heart Rate Zone

*Formula: THR Zone = estimated maximum heart rate X 65% and 90%*

*Estimated Maximum Heart Rate (MHR) = 220 - age*

MHR = 220 - Age = _____

MHR _____ X 65% (.65) = _____

MHR _____ X 90% (.90) = _____

---

***Target Heart Rate Zone =***

_____ Beats per minute to _____ Beats per minute

---

*Example: 32 year old petty officer*

*220 - 32 = 188*

*188 X .65 = 122*

*188 X .90 = 169*

*Target heart rate range is 122 - 169 beats per minute or 20-28 beat per 10 seconds.*

**Checking Your Exercise Pulse Rate**

You may be thinking, "How am I supposed to check my pulse while I am exercising?" It's simple. All you will need is a watch with a second hand. Count your pulse for 10 seconds and multiply by 6. Your pulse can be readily found in two places.

**Pulse Check Techniques**

## Table 8-5. Pulse Check Techniques

A carotid pulse can be found by running two fingers along the side of your neck from the back of your ear to the side of your Adam's apple.

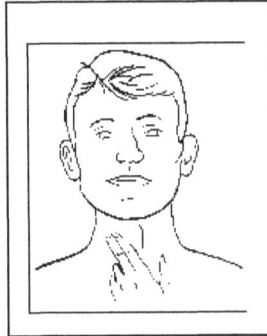

A radial pulse can be found by placing two fingers on the inside of your wrist, at the base of the thumb.

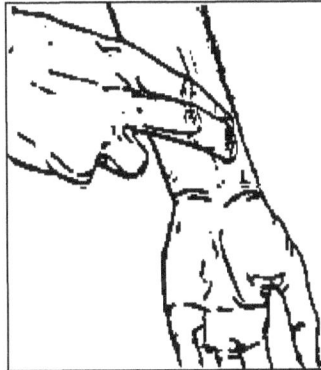

**Example:** A 32 year old petty officer has been jogging for 10 minutes. He wants to make sure that he is exercising in his zone. He stops jogging, counts his pulse for 10 seconds, and resumes jogging. He counted "23" beats, so he multiplies by "6" and gets 138 beats per minute which is his target zone.

Another way is to figure out your target heart rate and divide by "6" ahead of time. This way you don't have to multiply by "6" when exercising. If the 10-second count is low, speed up exercise, or if it is too high, slow down.

**Common
Questions on
Target Heart
Rate**

**Question:**

If exercise is supposed to be continuous, why do you stop to check your pulse?

**Answer:**

Most people cannot feel a pulse <u>and</u> exercise at the same time and often end up counting their feet hitting the ground instead. You may stop exercising for brief periods, as your heart rate will not drop significantly in the 15 seconds you stop. Remember to resume exercise as soon as you have counted.

**Question:**

What if the pulse rate for the individual was 195 beats per minute?

**Answer:**

They need to SLOW DOWN. If jogging, change to a brisk walk and recheck after a few minutes.

**Question:**

I can't jog for a full 30-40 minute period, but my heart rate doesn't get high enough by just walking. What should I do?

**Answer:**

Some people need to do a combination of walking and jogging. For instance, jog for 2 minutes, walk for 3 minutes, jog for 2 minutes, walk for 3 minutes, etc. After a person becomes more physically conditioned, a longer jogging period can be attempted with shorter walking periods. Remember to check heart rate periodically to monitor progress.

**Question:**

I don't think I can figure this out. This is too much of a bother. What should I do?

**Answer:**

It takes time to get used to checking your heart rate and at first you may feel silly. After daily practice, checking heart rate will become automatic with every physical training session. You might want to invest in a heart

**Common Questions on Target Heart Rate (cont.)**

rate monitor for simply keeping track of your daily heart rate during exercise. These are available at most sporting good stores and military exchanges. Talk with your Regional Health Promotion Manager about the details of Heart rate monitors.

Remember <u>you</u> are your own best judge when it comes to your exercise sessions. Some general rules:

1. *You should be able to carry on a conversation while exercising.*

2. *You should not be gasping for air during exercise.*

3. **Exercise should not leave you exhausted.**

## Barriers to Exercise

**"I Don't have the Time."**

The most common excuse for not exercising regularly is **no time**. Most people tend to find time for the things they enjoy. Does your work, family, travel, etc. prevent you from keeping up with your exercise goals? The key is to work in small amounts of exercise wherever we can. Although we have stressed that 40-45 minutes of aerobic activity is optimal for weight loss, other small bursts of physical activity add up and are relevant. They are not meant to replace cardiovascular conditioning, but do help by using calories. Let's illustrate this:

In 1980, a study done at the University of Pennsylvania School of Medicine observed the use of stairs vs. escalators in places where they were close to each other (i.e. subway stations, airports, and shopping malls). They found that overweight individuals were less likely to take the stairs. They also placed a poster at the bottom of the steps to remind people of the cardiovascular benefits of taking the stairs. The researchers found that twice as many lean individuals used the stairs after being reminded by the poster, while a small percentage of overweight individuals changed their habits even when reminded.

What does this tell us? It tells us that we can develop better habits in our lives to include "movement" in a society where everything we use is automated. How many times do you drive around the parking lot looking for that close space? Why not walk a little further? Do you live a few miles from work? How about riding a bike on good weather days? Think about ways to sneak exercise into your daily routine.

Don't let yourself be talked into common excuses. If these sound familiar to you, think about resolving your relationship with exercise. How important is it in your life? Why are you exercising? What do you expect exercise to do for you? What motivates you to exercise?

**It's Too Cold."**   Most of us live in variable climates, which can make it difficult to keep up our exercise routine. Trying to go out for your daily jog with overcast skies and temperatures in the low 30's can de-motivate even the most faithful runner. Keep in mind that you wouldn't avoid building a snowman, sledding, or snow skiing just because it was cold outside. You would just *dress appropriately*. The same holds true for exercise in cold weather.

The most important thing when exercising in the cold is proper cold weather attire. A rule of thumb is one light layer of clothing for every 10-15 degrees below 70°. Fabrics such as polypropylene absorb moisture while keeping you warm and dry. Cotton, on the other hand, gets wet and stays wet with perspiration. Polypropylene is best worn next to the skin under a waterproof, windproof outer layer such as Gore-Tex. If waterproof attire is not needed, a fabric such as fleece provides warmth without weight. A hat is essential in cold weather, as heat is rapidly lost from the head. Gloves or mittens made of wool, fleece, or polypropylene are also a necessity in cold temperatures. Consider exercising with a friend or shipmate. A buddy system can help in cold weather.

**It's Too Hot."**   If your average summer day is 89° and 90 % humidity by 9:00 am, then you have probably said "It's too hot" a few times. Hot weather can be very risky, even life-threatening if safety precautions are not followed. Dehydration and heat stroke are the primary concerns. Proper fluid intake is essential. Don't wait until you are dehydrated to increase your fluids. In addition to being well hydrated before you head out, you'll need 1/2 cup water replacement every 15 minutes.

Wear loose fitting, comfortable fabrics that are breathable such as cotton, and avoid dark colors. Wear only one layer of clothing such as a T-shirt and shorts. Exercising in a plastic suit is dangerous, as they cause profuse sweating and loss of vital fluid and prevent necessary cooling of the body.

Avoid exercising in the middle of the day when temperatures are the hottest. Plan your exercise in the early morning or evening. Pay attention to the various flags, black and red, which are flown to indicate heat index and to control physical activity. These flags indicate the wet bulb globe temperature (WBGT), an index of a combination of readings from three temperatures: dry, humid, and radiant heat. These three temperatures in combination provide a more accurate reading of heat stress intensity.

**Red flag** (WBGT of 88°-90°) indicates physical activity is advised only for members who have been working out in similar heat for a period of 2-6 weeks or more.

**It's Too Hot
(cont.)**

**Black flag** (WBGT of 90 °or higher) which indicates vigorous outdoor exercise, regardless of conditioning or heat acclimatization, is not advisable. In some areas of the country, hot humid conditions increase the risk from air pollution. No amount of acclimatization can make this safe.

Still too hot? Add water to your routine. Swimming and water-walking provide a cool alternative to hot weather. Another option is exercising in an air-conditioned gym or fitness center.

## Staying Motivated

**Adding Variety**

Many people find it hard to stay motivated and keep exercising. One reason may be boredom in doing the same exercise over and over on a daily basis. For example:

John uses the treadmill at the gym Monday, Wednesday, Thursday, and Friday for 25 minutes. He would like to do longer, but he is so bored, he decides to give up all together (or finds projects at work and home that prevent him from getting to the gym).

When it comes to exercise, variety is the key. Athletes call it cross-training. You may think, "but I'm not an athlete, how can I cross-train?" Cross-training is simply varying your routine to work different muscle groups as well as maintaining variety. For instance, running and cycling use the same muscles in different ways. Another example:

Susan jogs on Monday and Wednesday, does aerobics on Tuesday and Thursday and walks or bikes with her family on the weekends.

Being outdoors is a great way to vary your routine; jog or bike a different route. Top athletes vary their routines often to prevent the boredom that comes with repetition.

**What's the *Best*
Exercise?**

*It's the exercise you will do! In other words, it is one - or several - you are interested in and motivated to continue for a long period of time-A LIFETIME!*

## The Exercise Log

Much like keeping a dietary log, the exercise log is an important tool to keep track of your progress. (It is very hard on Friday to remember what you did on Monday!) This will allow you to look back over a week or

**Exercise Log (cont.)**

month's time to see your actual progress. Sample exercise logs are provided on the following pages. Make copies of these to record your progress.

**Guidelines to Determine Your FITT Exercise Plan**

It was stated at the beginning of this Chapter that a successful exercise plan incorporates each FITT component- *Frequency*, *Intensity*, *Type* of activity, and *Time* (length) of exercise.

The *Frequency* goal for exercise for weight loss is ***no less than 3 times per week,*** but research shows better results with 5 days a week of exercise. Refer to **Table 8-2** at the beginning of the chapter to determine the *Frequency* of weekly calorie expenditure.

**Cardio Exercise Log**

**Worksheet 8-1** helps you identify the *Type* of activity and *Time* needed to expend the required calories. **Worksheet 8-2** helps you determine the *Intensity* of aerobic activity. **Worksheet 8-3** on the following page will help you put together your comprehensive Cardio plan.

**Strength Training Log**

If you intend to start a weight training program don't forget to consult with trained personnel. They can get you started on a basic plan that will encompass all the FITT elements.

*Frequency* for strength training sessions should be 3-4 times per week if your goal is to build muscle mass. If combined with cardiorespiratory exercise, strive for 2-3 times per week. **Worksheet 8-4** will help you plan the *Intensity* & *Time* (determined by the number of repetitions and sets per exercise) and *Type* of exercises.

***Be sure to give each muscle group at least 48 hours rest between sessions.*** Strength training causes microscopic muscle tears (this is normal) and allows the muscle to grow. Rest allows the muscle to repair.

# Worksheet 8-3.  Aerobic Exercise Plan

*To establish your Aerobic Exercise Plan, calculate the following steps. Refer to the Tables and Worksheets earlier in this chapter to gather the information you need. Then transfer the data to the Chart.*

1. Frequency: # of days/week (*from Table 8-2*)      _____

2. Exercise Days of Week :  _____ _____ _____ _____ _____ _____

3. Calories expended per workout (*from Worksheet 8-1*)      _____

4. Intensity: THR Zone (*from Worksheet 8-2*)      _____

5. 10-Second THR Zone (*Step #4 divided by 6*)      _____

6. Exercise Time: minutes (*from Worksheet 8-1*)      _____

7. Type of Activity (*from Worksheet 8-1*)      _____

## *Aerobic Exercise Chart*

| *Exercise Factor* | *Sample Plan* | *My Plan* |
|---|---|---|
| 1. Frequency (# days/week) | 5 Days/Week | |
| 2. Exercise Days of Week | Mon.-Tues.-Wed.-Thurs.-Fri. | |
| 3. Calories expended per exercise session | 435 Calories | |
| 4. Intensity (THR Zone) bpm (beats per minute) | 122-169 bpm | |
| 5. 10 Sec. THR Range bpm (beats per minute) | 20-28 bpm | |
| 6. Time (min/ workout) | 30 min. | |
| 7. Type  of activity | Walk 15 min./mile | |

***Now, go to page 1-3 and complete Step8 on Worksheet 1-1, My Weight Management Plan.***

| Date | Aerobic Activity | Minutes | Miles | Perceived Exertion Level (6-20)* | Heart Rate | CALORIES BURNED |
|------|------------------|---------|-------|----------------------------------|------------|-----------------|
| | | | | | | |
| | | | | | | |
| | | | | | | |
| | | | | | | |
| | | | | | | |
| | | | | | | |
| | | | | | | |
| | | | | | | |
| | | | | | | |
| | | | | | | |
| | | | | | | |
| | | | | | | |
| | | | | | | |
| | | | | | | |
| | | | | | | |
| | | | | | | |
| | | | | | | |
| | | | | | | |
| | | | | | | |
| | | | | | | |
| | | | | | | |
| | | | | | | |
| | | | | | | |
| | | | | | | |
| | | | | | | |
| | | | | | | |
| | | | | | | |
| | | | | | | |
| | | | | | | |
| | | | | | | |
| | | | | | | |
| | | | | | | |
| | | | | | | |
| | | | | | | |
| | | | | | | |
| | | | | | | |
| | | | | | | |
| | | | | | | |
| | | | | | | |
| | | | | | | |
| | | | | | | |
| | | | | | | |

Worksheet 8-4

# Aerobic Training Log

Name:

* Perceived exertion levels on a scale of 6-20, 6 is very very light and 20 is very very hard.

# Worksheet 8-5: WEIGHT TRAINING EXERCISE RECORD

| Exercise | Machine # | Seat Position | Starting Weight | End of Week # ---------------- Weight #Reps/#Sets | End of Week # ---------------- Weight #Reps/#Sets | End of Week # ---------------- Weight #Reps/#Sets | End of Week # ---------------- Weight #Reps/#Sets |
|---|---|---|---|---|---|---|---|
| Leg Press | | | | _____ | _____ | _____ | _____ |
| Leg Curl | | | | _____ | _____ | _____ | _____ |
| Leg Ext | | | | _____ | _____ | _____ | _____ |
| Bench Press | | | | _____ | _____ | _____ | _____ |
| Incline Press | | | | _____ | _____ | _____ | _____ |
| Pec Dec | | | | _____ | _____ | _____ | _____ |
| Lat Pull down | | | | _____ | _____ | _____ | _____ |
| Rowing | | | | _____ | _____ | _____ | _____ |
| Arm Curls | | | | _____ | _____ | _____ | _____ |
| Triceps Curls | | | | _____ | _____ | _____ | _____ |
| Shoulder Press | | | | _____ | _____ | _____ | _____ |
| | | | | _____ | _____ | _____ | _____ |
| | | | | _____ | _____ | _____ | _____ |

Complete weight-training routine with a balanced abdominal and lower back workout routine.

Other methods of resistance training (other than weight training) can improve your strength and endurance. Examples are using your body weight as resistance, rubberized tubing, and partner-assisted exercises.

**Warm Up/Flexibility**: Perform an active warm-up for 5-10 minutes prior to lifting your first weight set; stretch muscles used between sets.

**Lifting Techniques**:
1. *Breathing* – exhale on the lift (positive); inhale on the release (negative).
2. *Counting* – 2 counts on the positive; pause: 1 second; 4 counts on the negative.
3. *Mechanics* - Never let the weight stacks touch during reps., or if lifting free weights, maintain slightly bent joints between reps.
4. *Posture* - Maintain correct body alignment throughout exercise sets.
5. *Frequency* - Lift a minimum of 3x/week, every other day – unless otherwise advised.

# Chapter 9

## LIFESTYLE CHANGES

## Overview

Lifestyle changes cannot be overlooked. Setting goals to make lifestyle changes helps you to stick with your plan, pay attention to your diet and, increase your physical activity.

Making changes in your lifestyle requires planning. First, identify thoughts, feelings, and behaviors that contribute to habits of overeating and lack of physical activity. You can replace negative thoughts, feelings, and behaviors with positive ones that will help you eat healthfully and exercise regularly for the rest of your life.

**Readiness to Change**

The first step is to become aware of how ready you are. There are many factors that determine your success at lifestyle change. You might have difficulties getting started, making a commitment, or setting realistic goals. On the other hand, while you might start out okay it may be a challenge to maintain motivation. In all, there are seven key factors that determine your readiness to change.

The following self-assessment is designed to help you understand the key factors that will influence your success at making the lifestyle changes.

**Readiness to Change**

# Worksheet 9-1. Readiness to Change Assessment

*Mark the box that indicates to what degree the statement best applies to your attitudes and beliefs about weight management. Answer every question.* Use this scale: *5= Always; 4= Almost Always; 3= Usually; 2= Sometimes; 1= Never*

*My Score*

| | |
|---|---|
| **A.** The decision to make this change is mine, rather than imposed by someone else. | |
| **B.** I have identified both the short term and long term benefits of my behavior change. | |
| **C.** I am not easily discouraged. | |
| **D.** I enjoy setting goals and then working to achieve them. | |
| **E.** I am good at keeping promises to myself. | |
| **F.** I like having a structure and schedule for my activities. | |
| **G.** I view my new behavior as a necessity, not an optional activity. | |
| **H.** My goals are realistic. | |
| **I.** Compared with previous attempts, I am more motivated now. | |
| **J.** I have a positive mental picture of my new behavior. | |
| **K.** Considering the outside stresses in my life, I feel confident I can stick to my program. | |
| **L.** I feel prepared for lapses and ups-&-downs in my behavior change program. | |
| **M.** I feel that my plan for behavior change is enjoyable and exciting. | |
| **N.** I feel comfortable telling other people about the behavior change I am making. | |
| **O.** I believe the benefits of the behavior change out-weigh the costs to change. | |
| **P.** I believe I am capable of managing my behavior. | |
| **Q.** I am confident I can say "no" to situations that would take me away from my goal. | |
| **R.** Once I set a goal, I think about it frequently. | |
| **S.** I am clear about the purpose of my behavior change. | |
| **T.** I am clear what information, skills, and support I need to change my behavior. | |
| **U.** Controlling my behavior is not a challenge to me. | |

**Calculate Your Score**

1. A + P + U = _____   2.  B + G + O = _____   3.  D + H + S = _____

4. C + I + M = _____   5.  J + L + R = _____   6.  E + K + Q = _____

7. F + N + T = _____

*Transfer each score Table 9-1 on the next page.*

**Factors Influencing Your Readiness to Change**

## Table 9-1. Factors Influencing Readiness to Change

| FACTOR | YOUR SCORE |
|---|---|
| 1. DECISION (A+P+U) | _____ |
| 2. VALUE (B+G+O) | _____ |
| 3. GOAL SETTING (D+H+S) | _____ |
| 4. MOTIVATION (C+I+M) | _____ |
| 5. MENTAL PREPARATION (J + L + R) | _____ |
| 6. COMMITMENT (E+K+Q) | _____ |
| 7. SUPPORT SYSTEM (F+N+T) | _____ |

**Interpretation**

Your score on each factor will range from 3 to 15. *Any score below 10 is low.*

*After you have calculated your score for each factor, circle any score below 10. These are the factors that need improvement. Follow the recommendations in the following section or develop your own strategies to prepare for lifestyle behavior change.*

## UNDERSTANDING THE FACTORS THAT AFFECT BEHAVIOR CHANGE

**Decision**

Take ownership and responsibility for the choices you make. Decisions are made two different ways. *Intrinsic* decisions are ones based on YOU. *Extrinsic* ones are imposed by others. Intrinsic decisions are long lasting because they are based on your personal values and beliefs. Responsible decisions are empowering because they are freely chosen. When planning your change, use self-empowering words such as " choose to, decide, want, can, will, my, mine."

**Values**

Your desired behavior change must have personal value. You should see benefits outweighing the challenges and sacrifices you will be making. A strong understanding of the purpose of the change is also necessary. Purpose means understanding how it fits or serves a bigger value, such as improved health or personal satisfaction. Take time to identify and write down your life's values and purposes. What is most important to you and how does this behavior change fit?

**Setting Goals**

Use the S.M.A.R.T. formula to set your goals (*see Worksheet 1-1*). Write your goals down and refer to them frequently. Since this is a process of refinement, be willing to modify and update your goals as you proceed. Make your goals work as road signs, letting you know where you are along the journey of behavior change. Be sure your goals are aligned with your purpose and your personal values.

**Motivation**

The inevitable "high" at the start of your behavior change can easily be followed by a "low"- characterized by burnout, low energy, and self-questioning of your goals. Be sure to identify and insert fun and play into your change plan. "Too much work and no play burns out almost anyone." Give yourself small rewards along the way. While feedback from others is important, don't allow it to determine your emotions or attitude towards your plan.

**Mental Preparation**

Successful performers regularly practice visualizing their goals. Instructional audiotapes that will take you through the visualization process can be helpful. Plan ahead for setback and lapses. They are inevitable, especially within the first six months. How you handle them will determine your success.

**Commitment**

Staying "on track" and sticking to your plan involves keeping your promise to yourself. If stress and distracting situations tend to get you "off track" then you need to implement a regular stress management routine. Time management and assertiveness skills also will assist you in staying "on track." Avoid the tendency to "give it all up" the first time you slip. Daily affirmations help keep your commitment strong.

**Support Systems**

Developing a system to successfully support your desired change involves several factors. This includes obtaining the information, skills, and help of others. Avoid stress and burnout by taking care of yourself -- physically, mentally, spiritually, and emotionally. Exercise, good nutrition, relaxation,

**Support
Systems (cont.)**

and healthy relationships at work and in your personal life will support your changes. A support group will put you in regular contact with people going through the same change. This provides moral support, change skills, and feedback on how you're doing. Confide in at least one close friend as your "sponsor" or mentor. Support systems for weight loss can even be found on the internet.

## Lifestyle Changes

This guide recognizes five *lifestyle factors* that influence weight management. They are:

    A. *Stress*

    B. *Self-talk*

    C. *Recognition & Reward*

    D. *Support Systems*

    E. *Assertiveness*

Making positive behavior changes in one or more of these areas can strongly support your weight management plan. Keep in mind that successful weight management implies *successful lifestyle management*. After you have considered each of the lifestyle factors, make a decision on which behaviors you want to change. **Worksheet 9-2** will help you do this.

**A. Stress
Management**

Stress is one of the major reasons why people overeat. You can, however, reduce stress-related overeating by learning to use methods other than food to cope with or reduce stress. The most common stress reduction techniques are deep breathing, deep muscle relaxation, visualization and forms of contemplative sitting - prayer, meditation, chanting, etc. Physical activity and exercise - including yoga - also are excellent stress reduction methods. You can apply some of these techniques on-the-spot as an alternative to misusing food.

### Deep Breathing

*You can do this almost anywhere and in almost any physical position. If possible, sit upright with feet on the floor and eyes closed*

    • Breath in slowly and fill up lungs and your diaphragm.

**Stress
Management
(cont.)**

- Inhalation should take 2-4 seconds. Feel your chest and diaphragm expand as they fill with air.

- Once you've achieved full inhalation hold this for 1-3 seconds.

- Upon exhalation, let go of all the physical, mental and emotional stress you carry.

- At the end of the exhalation hold this posture for 1-3 seconds.

- Repeat the cycle several times (3-15 minutes).

**Progressive Muscle Relaxation**

- Start by assuming a comfortable position - sitting or laying on your back.

- Close your eyes and take a few deep breaths.

- Starting with the muscles in the arches of your feet you will work up through the muscle groups of your body to your neck and face.

- Tighten each group of muscles and hold for 15 seconds. Then quickly release the tension. Repeat 1-2 times for each muscle group.

**Visualization**

- Select a quiet and relaxed environment. Turn down the lights.

- Assume a comfortable position.

- Take a few minutes to get yourself physically and mentally relaxed-use deep breathing.

- Keeping your eyes shut, drift away to a time or special place that you found to be calm, relaxing, and peaceful-the beach, a wooded area, the mountains, a field, etc.

- Let your imagination go and put yourself completely into this calm and peaceful environment.

**Stress Management (cont.)**

- Allow yourself to experience this scene with all your senses .- smells, touch, sounds, and even tastes.

- When you feel finished and relaxed, open your eyes, move your arms and legs, and swallow.

**B. Change Your Self-talk**

Negative thoughts can defeat even your best weight-loss intentions. The more aware you become of your negative thoughts, the better able you will be to stop them and replace them with supportive ideas that will ensure your success. For example, negative self-talk like, "It's no use!" "I'll never be able to do this!" can be replaced with, "This may be difficult, but I am a capable person who has done hard things before! I can do this!"

Sometimes we sabotage our own weight loss efforts by negative thoughts and feelings. If you recognize yourself in any of the following statements, take heed. Identifying behaviors is the first step to changing them.

**"I'm paying for it, so I might as well finish it"**

- If at a restaurant, ask for a doggie bag; if at home, wrap up the rest for leftovers.

- Is putting food into your mouth instead of down the disposal going to end world hunger?

**"I've already blown it today, so I'll start again tomorrow."**

- It takes 3,500 calories to gain a pound of fat

- Adding more calories is only going to make the situation worse

- Your body doesn't think in terms of days, but calories over a period of time

**"Just this once won't hurt."**

- Is this truly a rare occurrence, or is this more frequent than you would like to admit?

- How will you feel after eating-- is the guilt you may feel worth it?

**Self-talk (cont.)**

**"I feel so _____ (angry, stressed, bored, depressed, tired, etc.) and this food will make me feel better."**

- Evaluate what is causing the emotion and try techniques to deal with emotions without food (take a walk, play your favorite game, engage in a hobby, etc.).

- Food may temporarily be satisfying, but a binge may only add to feelings of guilt or depression.

**C. Recognize and Reward Success**

It is important to have short-term rewards while waiting for long-term effects. Referring to our example in Chapter 1, we set a goal of *five pounds of weight loss per month*. An example of a reward may be "I will buy a new pair of running shoes when I lose my first five pounds." Think about setting rewards when you set your short and long-term goals. You may even want to write them down. A reward does not need to involve spending money; you may want to do something you enjoy such as a leisurely afternoon in the park or sleeping in on a Saturday.

You can motivate yourself to continue on the road to weight loss by rewarding yourself for making good changes, and by obtaining the support of family and friends. For example, you can reward yourself with tickets to a concert, the theater, a movie, or weekend golf, resort, or spa trips that involve physical activities like hiking.

**D. Seek Support**

Consider where you can go for information, skills, instruction, and emotional support. A support person can be a spouse, a family member, friend, or shipmate. It needs to be someone who understands what you are going through or at least, has a desire to help you reach your goal. Join a support group or see a professional counselor. Fellow members can provide comfort and share ideas that can help you succeed.

You may want to use formal support groups available in the civilian community. Some are free of charge, while others range from a nominal fee to fairly expensive. Be careful of any weight loss plans or groups that charge a large amount of money. Paying money does not ensure results. There are also a variety of support groups that are free and can be accessed on the Internet. Check with your unit Health Promotion Coordinator or regional Health Promotion Manager for information on support groups in your area.

**E. Assert Your Needs**

Talk with your support person and others who have positive influence on your weight management behavior. Discuss what concerns you. It is essential to have open discussions about your plans and intentions.

**1. Communicate.** Sometimes we assume spouses or friends are "mind readers." Don't assume so. Instead let other know what you want. You may wish to say:

- "I'd prefer it if you wouldn't eat _____ in front of me."

- "I'd prefer if you wouldn't buy_____ from the grocery store."

- "I'd like for you to tell me when I am doing _____."

- "Would you exercise with me after work?"

- "If you bring in donuts for work, please leave them on your desk. I have a hard time resisting."

- "Please don't ask me to go to _____ for lunch. You know I have a hard time staying on my meal plan there."

**2. Speak up.** It's important - and doesn't hurt to ask for any of the following:

- Praise.

- Feedback- be specific with your needs.

- Cooperation and participation - shopping, exercising, cooking, meal planning, food cues.

- Support and encouragement.

- Gatherings that include activities and not just food.

- Minimize conversations about food.

- People not eat tempting food around you.

- Low-calorie food.

**Make Lifestyle Changes**

Now that you have looked at all five lifestyle factors that influence weight management you can put together a plan. **Worksheet 9-2** will help you identify the specific lifestyle changes you wish to make.

# Worksheet 9-2.  Make Lifestyle Changes

*Write down the specific lifestyle behaviors you want to make that support your weight management plan.*

A.  I will use the following *stress management techniques (what-when-where):*

_____

_____

B.  I will make these changes in my *self-talk (what-when-where)*:

_____

_____

C.  I will *recognize and reward my success (what-when-where?)*:

_____

_____

D.  I will obtain *support* from the following:

   1.  People:_____

_____

   2.  They will support me in the following way *(what & when)*:

_____

_____

E.  I will *communicate and assert* my needs *(what-when-where)*:

_____

_____

**_Now, go to page 1-3 and complete Step 9 on Worksheet 1-1, My Weight Management Plan._**

# Appendix A

# FREQUENTLY ASKED QUESTIONS

## Why do I always gain the weight back?

There is overwhelming evidence that humans have a constant weight range that they naturally maintain, and therefore, always return to. This is known as the set-point theory. It acts much in the same way that the human body returns to its own temperature level following illness.

Numerous studies have been done which support this theory. The most notable study involved "starved" volunteers who were given free access to food and allowed to eat ravenously until their weight returned to pre-diet level. The study showed that at that point appetite and calorie intake leveled off to pre-diet amounts. In another study, normal weight volunteers were deliberately placed on a diet to increase weight by 25 percent. They were then allowed to eat whatever they wanted. With no attempts to control their weight, they returned to their pre-diet weight levels.

It is this set-point that explains why dieters return to pre-diet weight once they stop restricting food intake. People may have different set-points throughout their lifetime, perhaps 125 pounds in their 20's, 150 pounds in their 40's, etc. It is believed many factors contribute to determining one's set-point. Factors such as metabolism and the number of fat cells may work together to "set" a level of weight that is normal for that person.

If all this sounds a little depressing, don't despair. It is believed that set-point can be changed by exercise. Exercise acts to increase resting metabolic rate, which means even when just sitting around, the body burns more calories. **The best predictor for who will lose weight and keep it off is people who make a lifelong commitment to regular exercise**.

## Is size and weight hereditary?

As the saying goes, "the apple doesn't fall far from the tree" is somewhat accurate when it comes to body type. The tendency to be overweight runs in families, and body type and fat distribution are to some degree a product of your genes. Since family members share environments as well as genes, it has been difficult to determine just how much influence heredity has on obesity.

**Hereditary Influences (cont.)**

Don't be discouraged if one or both of your parents are overweight. Although it may be more challenging due to your hereditary this does not mean you cannot control your weight by diet and exercise.

## Is it true that upper body fat is more dangerous than lower body fat?

Yes. Research shows that a person's risk of developing heart disease and diabetes is greatly increased when fat is distributed above the waist, verses in the abdominal area. Males tend to gain weight in the waist, which places them at greater risk. Females tend to gain weight below the waist.

Sometimes this is called the "apple" or the "pear" shape of the body. The apple shape is not exclusively male. The hormonal changes of menopause tend to cause a shift of weight from the hips to the waist.

## I want to stop smoking, but I'm afraid I'll put on even more weight. What should I do?

It's true that weight increase is associated with tobacco cessation- about four to six pounds, on average. Other factors associated with quitting tobacco - such as return of taste and smell for food - can result in increased calorie intake. Many smokers use tobacco as a stress reliever. When they quit, they often use food as a substitute. Smoking is a greater risk factor for death than being overweight, and therefore quitting should always be encouraged despite the small amount of weight gain. Once you have adjusted to your tobacco- free behavior, you can focus your efforts on healthy diet, exercise, and behavior change techniques.

## Does liposuction have a role in treating obesity or reducing body fat measurements?

By definition, liposuction is removal of fat under negative pressure, applied by means of a hollow suction tube tunneled through the subcutaneous fat by multiple small incisions.

Liposuction **is not** a treatment for obesity! The ideal candidate for liposuction is young and in good general health, with normal body weight and good skin tone.

While liposuction is available to active duty members at some naval hospitals, such cosmetic surgery is extremely restricted. In general,

**Liposuction (cont.)**

liposuction is limited to individuals who have localized areas of fat <u>despite</u> meeting height/weight standards. While liposuction may reduce waist and hip measurements somewhat, it is unlikely that a liposuction procedure would change a member's measurements from out of Coast Guard standards to within Coast Guard standards.

## I've been trying to lose weight for so long and nothing seems to work. What am I doing wrong?

When what you're doing isn't working, it is time to reevaluate your weight loss strategies. First, keep a food and exercise log. Write down everything that you eat after you eat it, **not** at the end of the day. Be sure to record your beverages. Hundreds of calories can be hidden in juices, sodas, and alcohol. Studies have shown that overweight people tend to *underestimate* food intake, and o*verestimate* exercise.

Check with your doctor to rule out medical causes as your problem with weight loss.

How is your meal spacing? Make sure you eat something low in fat within three hours of getting out of bed, and eat two more meals at 3-5 hour intervals after you get up. Routinely going without food for long periods of time can trick your body into believing food is scarce, and body fat stores must be conserved. We can easily handle a 12-14 hour fast when we are asleep.

Review your exercise log. Do you ***consistently*** follow your exercise plan? Remember, exercising only 3 days a week will ***maintain*** your current fitness. You need at least 4-5 days per week to optimize your fat-burning potential. How long are your exercise sessions. To burn body fat, you need aerobic exercise that works the large muscle groups, such as the thighs and buttocks. A longer duration and lower intensity workout may decrease the risk of injury and burn more calories. For weight loss purposes, it is the cumulative effect of exercise that burns calories.

## I hear sports and fitness supplements improve exercise performance. What is the Coast Guard's view on sports and fitness supplements?

There has been a rising popularity of supplement use in the Coast Guard. Coast Guard health promotion and medical professionals are concerned with the increased use of "sports and fitness" supplements sometimes referred to as ergogenic aids, among Coast Guard members. Webster's Medical Dictionary, 1995 Edition, defines ergogenic as "increasing the capacity for bodily or mental labor by eliminating fatigue symptoms." Industry-promoting ergogenic aids have many claims that these supplements improve physical performance. While some of the claims have some truth and supporting evidence to them, there are significant health and safety concerns for those using these supplements.

The "supplement industry" boom draws in 12 billion dollars a year. In 1994 federal legislation, the Dietary Supplement Health and Education Act passed a law to remove dietary supplements from FDA control after intensive lobbying by the supplement industry. Manufacturers now make broad statements in their ads and on their packages without the proof of safety and efficacy required for drug products. However, they can not make any specific medical claims such as "a supplement may be used to treat or prevent disease." Flawed studies are vigorously cited in support of dubious or even dangerous products. Unfortunately, manufacturers can make claims concerning the purity, safety, and efficacy of supplements to enhance performance without unbiased scientific evidence.

Individuals interested in weight loss, improving health, increasing muscular size or improving athletic performance have been tempted by the claims of these dietary supplements to help them attain their goals. When trying supplements, some individuals often feel stimulated or "energized," but this is often a "placebo affect." About 30% of people respond to a placebo sugar pill. Unfortunately, most of these supplements may not have any of the advertised effects on health or performance as promised by the manufacturer. Supplements may have negative and potentially fatal side effects, which include muscle cramping, diarrhea, headaches, tremors, stroke, heart attack, and seizures. The potential for injury or illness is high. Furthermore, there is no conclusive data that supplements help to build muscle or burn fat.

A recent article in the New England Journal of Medicine (December 21, 2000) concluded that the use of dietary supplements that contain ephedra alkaloids (sometimes called ma huang) pose a serious health risk to some users. Some of the serious health risks are adverse cardiovascular events, including heart attacks, high blood pressure, and death.

Because of the lack of FDA regulation on the food supplement industry, it is important for individuals to use extreme caution when taking supplements. Nutritional supplements are potent drugs and their dangers are not advertised. They can be marketed without the U.S. Food and Drug Administration review of safety or effectiveness, and many claims are unsubstantiated. The contents or concentration of active ingredients can differ remarkably from product to product due to the lack of regulatory control.

Scientific research repeatedly indicates that for both performance and health benefit, there is no "magic pill." Sound training principles, which include strenuous activity, healthy nutrition and adequate rest, result in both performance and health benefits. The following questions should be used to identify nutrition quackery:

Does it contain a secret ingredient?

**Supplements (cont.)**

Is the advertisement mostly case histories and testimonials?

Is it expensive?

Was any research actually performed?

Can a copy of the research be reproduced for review?

Where was it published?

Have the results been replicated by other researchers?

What kind of subjects were used?

Does it tell you not to trust others products?

To avoid nutrition quackery, the safest recommendation is to eat a well-balanced meal, exercise regularly, and rest for proper fuel supply to the body and mind. There is no magical secret to living a long, healthy life. The Coast Guard health promotion and medical professionals encourage everyone to eat well-balanced meals and exercise appropriately. Due to the lack of scientific evidence, supplements are not recommended for muscle building or fat burning.

## I've heard that different supplements can help you lose weight and improve muscle. Can you tell me anything about carnitine and chromium?

When it comes to nutritional supplements, there is always something new on the market being reported as the latest nutritional discovery. It is difficult for the average person to understand and sort supplement facts from fiction with the overwhelming amount of nutrition advice in the media today. In most cases, the nutrition claims for these supplements sound scientific and reasonable. However, there often isn't sound research to back the claims on most of the supplements! Carnitine is a compound synthesized in the body from glutamate and methionine. Carnitine (or L-carnitine) has been advertised as a "fat burner" that will improve cardiovascular function and muscle strength, and delay the onset of fatigue. Their claim is that carnitine increases fat utilization during exercise. No research supports increased use of fatty acids after carnitine ingestion, and no increase in performance has been demonstrated after its use.

Chromium is a mineral required for normal lipid and carbohydrate metabolism and assists insulin with carbohydrate and protein metabolism. Chromium acts as part of the glucose tolerance factor and may improve glucose tolerance in chromium-deficient patients.

Chromium is being sold in health food stores as chromium picolinate with claims that it will burn body fat while building muscle. Much of the

**Supplements (cont.)**

chromium hype is based on a few flawed studies which showed chromium improved muscle mass during strength training. Many well-controlled studies have been done in this area and have shown less promising results. In addition, there is no data to support the claim that chromium picolinate improves weight loss. More research is needed. While prescription medications undergo rigorous testing before approval, nutritional supplements do not. If the nutritional claim sounds too good to be true, it probably is!

Chromium is found in brewer's yeast, oysters, liver, and potatoes. Seafood, whole grains, cheese, chicken, meats, bran, fresh fruits and vegetables contain more moderate amounts.

Eating too many refined foods, such as white bread and sweets (which are low in chromium) may actually increase your need for chromium (to help process carbohydrates). A range of 50 to 200 micrograms has been designated as safe and adequate. While chromium content is difficult to measure in foods, most people get enough from the foods they eat. It is best to stick with food sources of chromium instead of a supplement. Getting too much chromium could hamper your absorption of iron and zinc. Be aware of nutritional supplements that claim quick and easy weight loss. The only thing getting smaller may be your wallet!

## I am taking birth control pills. Are these preventing me from losing weight?

Studies that have been done on women taking birth control pills show that some lose weight and some gain weight. Of course, if you start eating more or exercising less, you will gain weight regardless of whether you are taking the pill. Women who do gain weight despite watching their diet and keeping up with their exercise probably do so because of the slightly "anabolic" effect that some birth control pills can have. Although this is not to the extent seen in athletes who may take anabolic steroids to build muscle mass, one of the hormones in birth control pills may slightly increase muscle mass.

## I am going through menopause. Is this preventing me from losing weight?

Humans tend to gain weight as they age. This is due to a number of factors including a changing "set point," a change in muscle mass, a change in fat distribution and often a decrease in physical activity. Menopause generally occurs around the age of 50, which is the time when all of these factors come into play. This doesn't mean that you are

**Menopause (cont.)**

expected to get fat during menopause. A well-balanced, low-fat diet combined with regular exercise will allow you to maintain normal body weight throughout your life.

## I've heard a lot in the media recently about weight loss pills. Can these help me lose weight?

Dexfenfluramine is another drug that has just received FDA approval in the U.S., and has been approved for many years in other countries. FDA approval will expand the use of dexfenfluramine to long-term use. The medication is similar to fenfluramine (*fen-phen*) in both its actions on the brain and weight loss results. As with fen-phen, weight gain returns once patients stop taking it.

As with all medications, dexfenfluramine does involve some risks. A serious (but rare) side effect of primary pulmonary hypertension has been reported with dexfenfluramine use. Because of this, health officials in Europe have limited dexfenfluramine use to individuals who are at least 30 percent above desirable weight (those with significant health risks due to their obesity). To summarize, currently available medications available by a doctor's prescription will produce weight loss while taken, yet have some risk involved. Unfortunately, these medications have not been successful at producing permanent weight loss. The Coast Guard discourages the use of weight loss pills and they are not available in the clinics.

## I heard they discovered an "obese gene" in mice. Does this mean I can quit dieting?

Until recently, it was accepted that overeating was a character disorder and there was widespread belief that those who suffered from obesity simply lacked willpower. New knowledge of physiology, biochemistry, and genetics has led scientists to reexamine this accepted belief. It is no longer doubted that obesity is the consequence of both voluntary behavior and of defined and undefined metabolic factors.

Scientists have long recognized that some forms of obesity are hereditary, but the links between fat and genes remained a mystery until December 1994. That is when the obesity gene was discovered in mice. From that, a human obese gene was cloned. Found in fat cells, the obese gene makes a protein "message" that travels via the bloodstream to the brain and says "I've had enough food, stop eating." In the strain of obese mice that were studied, the protein message is mutated and the message never gets to the brain. Since the principle action of this protein is to make the animal thin, researchers have named this obese gene "leptin" from the Greek root Leptos meaning thin. Grossly obese mice were given daily injections of leptin, and after one month, food intake and body weight dropped by 50 percent.

As encouraging as these results are, they don't necessarily translate to obese humans (keep in mind that while mice "feed", humans dine, celebrate, feast, etc.). Early studies done with the obese human gene suggest that the common forms of human obesity aren't due to anything as simple as a flaw in the obese gene. Obesity in humans is due to many factors, both environmental and genetic.

Because of this, researchers had to find mice (with obesity traits) that more closely resemble obesity in humans. They found a strain of mice that grow plump when their diet contains too much fat. After fattening up the mice, researchers injected them with leptin. In response to the leptin, the mice ate less high fat food and lost weight. However there is another strain of obese mice that are resistant to leptin. What this suggests is that there are probably various types of obesity in humans. Research is now focusing on the brain to determine why the message to stop eating is not getting through despite the presence of leptin in fat cells.

Much work needs to be done before considering drug therapy with leptin in humans. First, researchers need to establish safety of leptin in animals. If leptin is found to be safe, there will be a problem with drug delivery. Since leptin is a protein, it would be destroyed in the digestive tract. It would therefore have to be injected, probably daily, much in the same way insulin must be injected. Although many people probably wouldn't mind daily injections to control their obesity, human testing is still years away.

While all this new science may seem like a "cure" for obesity, any potential treatments with drugs or genes must be **in addition** to diet and exercise. Reducing body fat with leptin while eating a high-fat diet will carry its own health risks. One interesting note: researchers found that diet and exercise help the brain respond to leptin.

Many people ask the question, "if this is a mutation in a gene, why are we seeing the increase in obesity as compared to 50 years ago?" The theory is that this is not a sudden mutation, but that it has always been there. These were our "survival genes" for times when food was scarce. Now that we are surrounded by an abundance of high-fat foods and have a sedentary lifestyle, these genes make it easier for us to gain weight and store body fat. Maintaining a healthy diet and an active lifestyle are the best defenses for preventing obesity.

# What is meant by a "Low Fat" Food?

A "low-fat" food is one which contains 3 grams of fat or less per serving. Low fat milk (or 2 percent milk) contains 5 grams of fat per serving. At the present time, milk is exempt from food labeling laws. That may change soon as the Food and Drug Administration (FDA) is proposing eliminating the standards of identity for low fat and skim milk products. Under the proposal, milk products containing 1.5 %to 2 % milk fat could no longer use the term "low-fat", but instead could be called "reduced-fat milk". Milk containing 1 % milk fat could be labeled "low-fat milk" (it contains 1.5 grams of fat per serving).

# Appendix B

# HEALTHY COOKING TECHNIQUES

## Recipe Modifications

| *When a Recipe Calls For:* | *Choose These Instead* |
|---|---|
| Regular ground beef | Extra-lean ground beef/ ground turkey |
| Baking chocolate 1 oz | 3 Tbs. powdered cocoa plus 1 Tbs. oil |
| Meat Juice for gravy | Skim or pour off fat first |
| Spaghetti sauce | Homemade - omit the oil; Store bought - reduced fat |
| Marinating meat | Use wine, fruit juices or broth instead of drippings |
| Oil in baking | Use applesauce instead for muffins |
| 1 whole egg | $^{1}/_{2}$ cup egg substitute or 2 egg whites |
| 1 cup butter | 1 cup soft margarine |
| 1 cup solid vegetable shortening | $^{3}/_{4}$ cup liquid vegetable oil |
| 1 cup whole milk | 1 cup skim milk |
| 1 cup heavy cream | 1 cup evaporated skim milk |
| 1 cup sour cream | 1 cup non-fat plain yogurt or 1 cup non-fat cottage cheese whipped in a blender to a smooth consistency |
| 1 oz regular cheese | 1 oz low fat/non-fat cheese |
| 8 oz cream cheese | 8 oz low fat/non-fat cream cheese or eat half the normal amount |
| 2 slices bacon | 1 Tbs. imitation bacon bits or 1 oz lean ham |
| 1 Tbs. mayonnaise | 1 Tbs. low fat/non-fat mayonnaise or 1 Tbs. plain low fat yogurt |

# Low-fat Cooking Substitutions

| When a recipe calls for: | Substitute: |
| --- | --- |
| 1 whole egg | 1/4 c egg substitute or 2egg whites |
| 1c shortening or butter (baking) | 3/4 c liquid oil or 1 c margarine (2 sticks) |
| 1 tbsp. oil/butter (sautéing) | 2 tbsp. broth or wine, or 1 tsp. oil with no-stick spray, or diet margarine |
| 1 tbsp. shortening or butter | 2 tsp. liquid or 1 tbsp. margarine or 1 tbsp. diet margarine |
| 1 square chocolate (1 oz.) | 1 tbsp. dry cocoa powder + 1/2 tbsp. liquid oil |
| 1 tbsp. butter (seasoning) | 1 tbsp. reduced-fat margarine or fat free margarine |
| 1 c whole milk or cream | 1 c skim milk or 1 c skim evaporated milk |
| 1 c sour cream | 1 c nonfat yogurt or fat-free or low-fat cottage cheese or 1 c nonfat sour cream (blended) |
| 1 oz. cream cheese | 1 oz. low-fat cottage cheese (blended) or 1 oz. fat-free or low fat cottage cheese |
| 1/4 c oil (baking) | 2 tbsp. oil + 2 tbsp. nonfat yogurt or 1/4 applesauce or banana strained fruit or non fat yogurt |
| 1 egg + 3 tbsp. oil (baking) | 1/2 c nonfat yogurt |
| 1 tbsp. mayonnaise | 1 tbsp. fat-free or reduced-fat mayonnaise or 2 tbsp. non fat yogurt |
| 1 c cream soup | 1 c reduced-fat cream soup |
| 1 oz. cheese | 1 oz. reduced-fat or fat-free cheese, or 3/4 oz regular cheese |
| 1/2 c nuts | 1/2 c Grapenuts or omit entirely |
| salad dressing & condiments | non-fat & low sodium substitutes |
| evaporated milk | evaporated *skim* milk |
| sugar | sweet flavors-vanilla, cinnamon, almond or reduce sugar by 1/4/-1/3 without affecting results |
| vegetable dips | non-fat yogurt & seasoning |

# Sample Low-fat Cooking Methods

- Use non-stick pots and pans. This enables you to use little or no added fat.

- Steam or sauté vegetables.

- Use a light coat of a vegetable oil spray. Choose olive or canola oils instead of using leftover bacon grease, lard, vegetable fat, etc.

- Experiment with nonfat liquids, such as Worcestershire, chicken broth or tomato juice.

- Poach poultry and fish.

- Trim off all visible fat from meat and remove the skin from chicken.

- Broil or bake meats, poultry, and fish instead of frying them.

- For stewing or soups, cook the meat ahead of time, let cool and skim off the accumulated fat before you go on.

- Eat more fish, white poultry and veal, avoid cuts of high-fat (marbled) red meat.

- Use water-packed tuna and salmon rather than oil-packed fish.

- Make gravies with fat-free broth, skim milk and cornstarch.

- Prepare vegetables with seasonings or lemon juice rather than fat-containing sauces.

- Use fat-free broth to cook vegetables instead of sautéing them.

- Serve foods simply, without added sauces.

- Reduce fat in recipes by 1/2 without affecting the final product.

- Select fresh fruit as substitutes for sweet desserts.

# Appendix C

# FOOD LABEL TERMS AND DEFINITIONS

---

**"Free"**        The product contains no amount (or physiologically inconsequential), of one of these components: fat, saturated fat, cholesterol, sodium, sugars, or calories. For instance, "fat free" means less than 0.5 grams per serving and "calorie free" means less that 5 calories per serving.

**"Low"**         This food could be eaten frequently without exceeding dietary guidelines for one or more of the following components: fat, saturated fat, cholesterol, sodium, and calories. The following terms apply:

| | |
|---|---|
| **Low fat** | 3 grams or less per serving |
| **Low saturated fat** | 1 gram or less per serving |
| **Low sodium** | Less than 140 mgs per serving |
| **Very low sodium** | Less than 35 mgs per serving |
| **Low cholesterol** | Less than 20 mgs per serving |
| **Low calorie** | 40 calories or less per serving |

**"Lean"**        Less than 10 grams of fat, less than 4 grams of saturated fat, and less than 95 mgs of cholesterol per serving and per 100 grams.

**"Extra Lean"**  Less than 5 grams of fat, less than 2 grams of saturated fat, and less than 95 mgs of cholesterol per serving and per 100 grams.

**"High"**        One serving of the food contains *20 percent or more* of the Daily Value for a particular nutrient.

**"Good Source"** One serving of the food contains *10 percent to 19 percent* of the daily value for a particular nutrient.

**"Reduced"**     A nutritionally altered product containing *25 percent less* of a nutrient or of calories than the regular product does.

**Less"**　　A food, whether altered or not, *contains 25 percent less* of a nutrient or of calories than the reference food.

**Light"**　　A nutritionally altered product *contains one-third fewer* calories *or half of the fat* of the reference food, or the sodium content of the low-calorie, low-fat food has been reduced by 50 percent.

**More"**　　One serving of the food, altered or not, contains a nutrient in a quantity that is *at least 10 percent* of the Daily Value more than the reference food.

# Appendix D

# REFERENCES

*The American Dietetic Association's Food & Nutrition Guide*, Duyff, Roberta, Chronimed Publishing (1996).

*The Balancing Act*, Kostas, Georgia, Quebecor Pertaining Book Group (1998).

*Coast Guard Wellness Manual*, COMDTINST M6200.1 (1997).

*Fit & Well*, Fahey, Insel, and Roth, Mayfield Publishing (1999).

*Mayo Clinic Healthy Weight Plan*, Mayo Clinic (1998).

*Nutrition and Weight Control Self-Study Guide,* U.S. Navy NAVPERS 15602A (1996).

*Peak Performance Through Nutrition and Exercise*, Singh Anita, Tamara Bennett and Patricia Deuster, Uniformed Services University of the Health Sciences F. Edward Herbert School of Medicine (1999).